Baking

Bun in the Oven

A Recipe Guide for Parents to Creating a Healthy Baby from Pre-Conception through the First Year

Rhian Young, ND

This book is dedicated to my children who I learned from by nature of walking through these precious days, my husband who puts up with my insistence on a healthy diet and environment, my staff who held down the fort while I took time off to write this book and of course my loyal patients who I learn from every day and become a better doctor, a better investigator and a better teacher.

Many blessings to all who read this book, for you, your children, your grandchildren and any person that you could possibly make even a small improvement in their life by reading and sharing this information.

--Dr. Young

TABLE OF CONTENTS

INTRODUCTION

I decided to write this book because, just like every mom, I think my babies are perfect! If you are already a parent, you will know that is just a given. That aside, I feel passionate about what we, as mothers (and fathers!) do before conception, during incubation and for one year after birth. Those two years (give or take) are the ONLY two years of your baby's entire life that you have complete control over what goes into them and what sort of environment they "bake" in and what "ingredients" they are given to accomplish the ultimate goal of optimal development. If we choose to embark on the adventure of parenthood, it is a huge sacrifice from day one and it will begin a lifetime of sacrificing for our children. Those two years are the ultimate time of sacrifice and a precious gift you can give your baby and bank on the fact that for the rest of their life, you provided something that they will cherish.

If you are already pregnant, I want you to read this and focus on the fact that you only now have all of the information you need. Try as hard as you can to not anguish on what you *could* have done, *should* have done and/or didn't do. Do not ruminate on it and punish yourself. If you don't already, now is the time to start living looking forward and throw away the rear-view mirror. I always say that the decisions we make are the best decisions at the moment we made them with all the facts we had at the time. How could you have done anything different if you didn't actually KNOW you were pregnant? How could you have known what to do at the time because you hadn't been blessed with the knowledge that is going to come to you? So, move forward and do the best you can from this point on.

I originally intended to write this book in sections and recommend that if you were already pregnant, to move to the section that was just on pregnancy and the first year but as I started writing, I realized that every piece of information in this book is imperative for every step of the process. It cannot be broken down. There are some parts that are more important at certain phases but none can be excluded at any phase in the pre-conception, pregnancy and breastfeeding part of the journey. So, read on, regardless of where you are at because this knowledge will help you improve your health for the rest of your life, in addition to helping you "bake the perfect bun".

SECTION 1

PLANNING THE RECIPE

Planning is an imperative part of any good culinary masterpiece. If you have the opportunity to plan ahead of time, you have a huge advantage over those who don't. If you are already pregnant, it means it is all the more important to get down to business of getting these things done.

When planning, you need to address some core issues with your significant other. In my line of work, we treat the whole person, mind, body and spirit. How can these aspects of the individual really be differentiated as they mesh together like sifting the dry ingredients of your favorite quick bread? They can, however, be somewhat isolated as we start to break things down one ingredient at a time.

CHAPTER 1

RELATIONSHIP PREPAREDNESS

As a couple, you and your partner, the two creators of your baking masterpiece, can start by working on your relationship. It is important to be on the same page as you prepare to change your life in ways that you will only understand once you walk through it. People can tell you 100 different ways how much your life will change but you cannot fully understand the magnitude of that change until you live it. It is best to prepare by planning a sit down talk to go through some of the hard questions. I recommend that you answer these questions separately then come together to discuss your answers. Having your answers prepared individually will give you the clearest picture of the first instinct answers you each have so you are not swayed by the other in how you really feel.

Questions to ask yourself and have your partner answer and discuss together:

1. Are you both ready to make a baby? If not, what is holding you back? If your hesitations are tangible things, can you make a plan on how you can get through those hurdles or accomplish those goals or realize those dreams so that you can be in a place of preparedness for the next phase in your life?
2. Are you financially stable? How will your finances be supported after the baby comes? Consider

planning a budget with baby supplies, food, initial startup costs (nursery items in particular), etc. to avoid any surprises and thus avoid any conflict with your spouse. Always leave room for a little extra. It is better to spend less than you planned versus more and be in over your head.

3. Will you or dad stay home with the baby? If not, who will take care of the baby while you work? Are you both in agreement with that plan?
4. Is your relationship strong enough to endure the changes that will occur when you are pregnant and even more so when the baby comes? What are your hobbies and what do you like to do together? If you are not able to do those things, how will your relationship change? What are some alternative activities you can do for fun?
5. Does your current living situation lend itself to adding a human being? If not, what do you think is a feasible plan to make accommodations for a baby?
6. What are your expectations of each other when it comes time to take care of the baby? Will it be 50/50? Will you take turns at night? Who will be the primary caregiver? Will you both attend well-baby visits? Will you make decisions together regarding care?
7. Will the baby sleep with you? In your bed? In your room in his/her own bed? Or in his/her own room in the crib?

8. What is your parenting style? What is acceptable punishment? If one of you believes in spanking and the other considers that abuse then you will end up fighting. Coming to an agreement early on will spare you the future heartache.
9. How do you each see your life changing as a couple? Your whole world will revolve around the baby's needs for a good amount of time. Some people think that nothing will change—you'll just keep doing what you are doing, just with a baby in tow and a car seat in the back. This is not usually how it ends up playing out. Talk to some friends and make a plan, or at minimum, come to an agreement that you will be open to seeing what life brings.
10. Will you still travel? If you are jet setters, you will find traveling changes tremendously. Set some expectations now so that one or both of you are not disappointed.
11. Will you have date nights? If one of you thinks you are going to still go out every Friday night alone as a couple and the other thinks you will go out once a month or worse, every 3 months, someone is going to become frustrated. Open the lines of communication regarding things like this and don't forget to reference question #2 because babysitters are expensive, especially for infants!

12. How will you maintain intimacy? Same as date nights—know your partner's expectations and vice versa to avoid disappointment and conflict.
13. Will your work schedules change? If you will both be working, are you able and willing to adjust your schedules to accommodate a small child? If not, are you ok with what that looks like?
14. How many kids do you want? How close together? I know, I know, if you haven't even gotten to baby number one yet, how can you think about the next one? But it is important to have that conversation. In reality, you should have had that conversation before you said your vows if you are already married. But if you haven't, do it now. It could also change how you approach things—if you know you are only having one then it can change how you go about decorating the nursery (maybe not wise to buy baseball or butterflies so that you can reuse things for the second baby) or how you plan your finances or what decisions you make about your career.

These are all vital questions to ask. If you disagree strongly with any of these things, you need to work toward a resolution before you get pregnant as these things left unanswered can create stress in the relationship and therefore stress in your body. Your body will be under enough stress so eliminating potential conflict and obstacles whenever possible is a great first step, especially in your relationship.

CHAPTER 2

INDIVIDUAL PREPAREDNESS

Now that we have the relationship issues covered, let's talk about you as an individual.

Do you feel that you are strong enough in your own mind and spirit? As your body goes through the many, many changes from conception to growth to delivery and after, can you manage those changes? Are you suffering from any chronic emotional turmoil? Consider trying to find peace with those things so that you don't end up having to deal with severe depression or anxiety while you are pregnant or after the baby is born. Dealing with these things now will help prevent post-partum depression.

If you are on medication to deal with depression or anxiety, you need to work on getting off the medications. It is best to work with someone who is supportive of alternatives. There are many other ways to treat depression and anxiety and I could probably write a whole additional book on this subject. Again, in a perfect world, these things would be dealt with before you ever become pregnant. Finding the CAUSE of these things is often the best way to get off medications. It could be something simple like vitamin D deficiency or not eating a balance diet or not getting enough exercise or sleep. We will address these things in the next few pages.

Are you prepared to face the physical changes that your body will endure as you lose your current figure and have to look at a newly revised version of yourself in the mirror every day? If this is an area you already struggle with, it will get worse as the weight comes on and even more so after the baby is born. It is best to communicate with friends or family or your partner about your insecurities and negative feelings. Also, make a plan about how you are going to deal with it—will you continue to exercise through pregnancy, will you work to get back to your regular routine after the baby is born? These are issues and details that you should think about and plan for in advance, so that in the moment, you don't lose yourself to the negative messages that will inevitably play in your head.

Managing stress is key to preparing your mind, body and spirit/soul. Recent research says that stress may contribute to 30% of infertility issues according to WebMD. Stress can interfere with our hormones thus making conception a challenge, or worse, impossible. In today's world, we have different stressors but our bodies perceive stress the same way they did thousands of years ago. It is in our DNA to not be able to conceive during times of extreme stress. This genetically programmed regulatory system was a way to preserve our species. If babies were born during times of drought or famine or if the mother was unable to do what was required to survive, then babies would not survive. Our system is programmed to recognize stress and shut down the proper messaging system to allow for conception. The point is—if you really want to try to have a baby, find a way to create more harmony and manage your stress. (WebMD, n.d.)

SECTION 2

PREPARING THE "KITCHEN" (aka The Body)

Anyone who has ever cooked something that doesn't just come out of a box knows you don't just dive in without making sure you have all the ingredients. Of course, you also want to make sure your kitchen is ready for the task of cooking such as clean counter tops, an empty sink, etc. When it comes to the business of making babies, ideally, your body needs to be "cleaned" in preparation. Some people like to do this a year in advance, others like to do it two weeks before ovulation. Of course, the longer ahead you can do it, if you can maintain it, the better it will be for both you and the baby. What people often fail to remember is that the eggs that we have in our ovaries are genetic material. All genetic material is subject to mutation and can be altered by environmental and nutritional exposures and choices we make. So keeping your eggs healthy is extremely important. This concept also applies to your partner. This is one of the precious time frames that DAD can actually contribute to this "time of sacrifice". In an ideal world, both parents would work together to "prepare the kitchen", at least one year in advance.

Preparing the "Body" is definitely the biggest driving factor as to why you likely picked up this book to begin with. People like to skip the mind/spirit stuff because it is too hard or too intangible but before we move on, I want to say that managing stress has been one of the biggest factors in the women I have helped get pregnant. Now I will move on...many women ask me how they can help their body to get ready for pregnancy. A lot of the answers you will read here are probably things you already know but need to hear it one more time now that you are truly ready to embark on this journey.

CHAPTER 3

MEDICATIONS

If you are currently on medication, it would be best to find alternatives to work to rid your body of the pharmaceuticals as many of them can have a detrimental effect on the fetus. Even if they claim not to, if something was wrong with your baby, wouldn't you always wonder if it was the medication you were on? Sometimes we turn to medications because it is the easiest or quickest route to deal with our problems. But the game is changing...this time is no longer about YOU, it is about your baby (within reason of course).

On the flip side, if you are on a medication that is required to keep you safe medically, be sure to discuss with your doctor if there are other options that will treat your condition with the least potential to cause harm. Sometimes older versions of a similar medication have a longer track record and may be a safer alternative to a newer drug.

You can look up your drug on various websites. The FDA has created a list based on animal studies and of course human reports after the fact. Here are the general guidelines for drug safety:

CLASS	EXPLANATION	EXAMPLES
Class A:	No known risk factors or evidence of harm to baby	Levothyroxine, Liothyronine, magnesium sulfate
Class B:	No risks shown in animal studies. No studies performed on humans or no data showing adverse effects in human children.	Metformin, HCTZ, Cyclobenzaprine, Amoxicillin, Pantoprazole
Class C:	Animal studies show harm to fetus. No studies performed on humans or no data showing adverse effects in human children.	Tramadol, Gabapentin, Amlodipine, Trazodone, Prednisone
Class D:	Definitive risk and harm to fetus but in cases where the mother requires the medication to keep her safe or alive, the benefits outweigh the risks.	Lisinopril, Alprazolam, Clonazepam, Lorazepam, Losartan, Topamax
Class X:	Definitive risk and harm to a significant degree and thus contraindicated in pregnancy or people who may become pregnant.	Atorvastatin, Simvastatin, Warfarin, Methotrexate Finateride

There are many resources online to help you determine if your medication is safe so that you have all the information when you go to speak to your doctor.

(www.FDA.com, n.d.) (American Pregnancy Association, n.d.) (Drugs.com, n.d.)

CHAPTER 4

BALANCING FEMALE HORMONES

Let me assure you that if you have issues with your cycle such as PMS, heavy bleeding, acne, severe cramping, etc. then you likely have a hormonal imbalance. You should seek out a provider that will do a full panel of blood work in two phases of your cycle. What that means is that on day 1 (the first day of your period), you start what is called the follicular phase and this lasts approximately 2 weeks. After ovulation, you begin the luteal phase. Most people have approximately a 28 day cycle (plus or minus 3 days). It is a good idea to have your hormones checked around day 7 and around day 21 so that you know what your hormonal status is in order to optimally prepare your body. If your hormones are significantly out of whack, you may have trouble conceiving or worse, conceive fine but lose the baby after a few weeks of conception due to insufficient progesterone. Each hormone involved in the female cycle has a role to play in helping you become pregnant. Here is the breakdown of what function they have in the body:

HORMONE	SOURCE	ACTION/ ROLE	CONSEQUENCE OF IMBALANCE
ESTROGEN (Estradiol)	Ovaries & Follicles	Changes cervical mucous to help sperm survive	High estrogen or estrogen dominance can suppress FSH.

		Signals release of LH Helps the lining of the uterus grow Increases blood flow during pregnancy	Low estrogen can prevent proper cervical changes for sperm and may not allow for LH release.
PROGES-TERONE	Ovaries Corpus Luteum	Maintains the uterine lining to allow fertilized egg to implant Later in pregnancy, it softens cartilage in preparation for birth	Low progesterone will result in miscarriage or inability for the egg to implant. High Progesterone is not typically detrimental to fertility
FSH—Follicle Stimulating Hormone	Pituitary gland in the brain	Signals the ovary to make a follicle	If too high, it may indicate the ovaries are not functioning If too low, it

			may indicate eggs are not being made or there is a significant amount of stress or the pituitary gland is not functioning
LH—Luteinizing Hormone	Pituitary gland in the brain	Signals release of the egg from the follicle	If too high or too low, ovulation does not occur
TESTOS-TERONE	Ovaries Adrenal glands	Prevent follicles from dying too early	If too high, causes irregular or absent menses If too low, follicles may die before maturation
DHEA-SULFATE	Adrenal glands	Precursor to other hormones	High or low levels may cause hormone imbalance and interfere with the normal hormone processes and

			their role & function

(Hormones that Play a Role in Conception, n.d.)

(Women Fitness, n.d.) (What to Expect, n.d.) (Science Daily, n.d.)

(WebMD, n.d.) (Women to Woment, n.d.)

You now have a list of the hormones that should be checked by your provider when you are in the process of getting ready to conceive. Should any of these be "off", it will be time to prepare your body through supplementation. We will discuss this in the upcoming sections.

To recap, request the following hormone blood tests from your physician:

1. Estradiol
2. Progesterone
3. FSH
4. LH
5. Testosterone
6. DHEA-Sulfate

CHAPTER 5

THYROID

Thyroid function is another thing to consider. It is also a hormone and plays a role in fertility. Your thyroid is often referred to as the "master gland" as it regulates most of the other hormones along with metabolism, brain function, heart function, lung function, bowel function, skin function, temperature regulation, cholesterol balance, etc. Most organs in the body have receptors for thyroid hormone.

Although science can't explain a biological reason, if your thyroid is not functioning optimally, you may have trouble conceiving. Research now shows that low thyroid, even sub-clinical hypothyroid can have an effect on the baby's brain development. Sub-clinical hypothyroidism is where the numbers are falling close to the normal range or very slightly elevated TSH with normal free (circulating) hormone levels. These patients usually have mild symptoms. Symptoms of low thyroid are vast but some of the main issues include fatigue, inability to lose weight despite adequate effort, dry skin, constipation, and depression.

Low thyroid function during pregnancy can cause the following issues:

1. Anemia—low red cells which can lead to fatigue, shortness of breath, restless leg and other issues
2. Myopathy—muscle weakness and muscle pain

3. Congestive Heart Failure
4. Pre-Eclampsia—a serious increase in blood pressure than can lead to emergency delivery of the baby
5. Placental abnormalities—which can put the baby at risk for improper development and death
6. Post-Partum hemorrhage—one of the leading causes of pregnancy related deaths.
7. Still Birth—death in the womb
8. Miscarriage
9. Low birth weight
10. Multiple long-term effects on the baby.

There is also a potential for elevated thyroid function or hyperthyroid. This usually presents in the form of Grave's disease and occurs in 1 in 1500 pregnancies which can result in death of the baby in some cases and in others, elevated heart rate, small size and even physical malformations. Uncontrolled hyperthyroidism during pregnancy can cause several complications, similar to that of hypothyroidism. They are slightly different but include:

1. Pre-Eclampsia
2. Congestive Heart Failure
3. Thyroid Storm
4. Low birth weight
5. Premature delivery
6. Death of baby & miscarriage

It is also important to note that thyroid levels are affected by estrogen and Hcg levels once you are pregnant. Monitoring the thyroid throughout pregnancy is equally important (more to come on this in the next section).

So, as you can see, making sure the thyroid is functioning optimally is critical prior to conception when possible.

(american thyroid association, n.d.)

(NIH, 2012)

CHAPTER 6

ENVIRONMENTAL EXPOSURES

This section will probably be one of the more alarming and eye-opening sections for a lot of people. Most of us go about our daily lives, blissfully unaware that we are being poisoned or worse, poisoning ourselves. There isn't much we can do about the air we breathe other than move away from where you currently live and go to the mountains. That is obviously not practical and of course, would be bordering on neurotically cautious to make such drastic decision based on wanting to get pregnant. You can control the air in your house and the chemicals you use in your house and of course the things you ingest, the water you drink and the products you use on your skin. I am going to go through a list of items and products and discuss the potential adverse effects they may have on your body or on your developing baby.

Since we are discussing the pre-pregnancy stage, it is important to start with a list of "endocrine disruptors". These are chemicals that literally affect your hormones and thus your ability to get pregnant and will usually affect a growing baby as well.

They interfere with your endocrine system in three possible ways:

1. They structurally mimic your hormones. This means they bind to your hormone receptors and thus

increase your hormone levels to an artificially toxic level.

2. They bind to the normal receptor and block your natural hormones from binding. This prevents your body from being able to function properly.
3. They interfere with the normal production of hormones. As a result, the body doesn't have what it needs to function properly.

(National Institute of Environmental Health Sciences, n.d.)

ENDOCRINE DISRUPTORS:

THE CHEM-ICAL	WHERE IT IS FOUND / WHAT TO AVOID	EFFECTS ON THE BODY	EFFECTS ON BABY
BPA	Lines cans of canned foods Thermal paper from receipts Plastics with "PC" on them Plastics with #7	Breast cancer Infertility Obesity Heart disease	Affects the brain, behavior, prostate gland of the fetus Also causes same effects in children later when continually

			exposed Early onset puberty
ATRAZINE	Herbicide, used mostly on corn crops Tap water (due to run off)	Breast cancer Prostate inflammation & possible prostate cancer	Delayed puberty
DDT	Pesticide	Causes infertility	Damages reproductive organs causing infertility later in life Increases risk of childhood obesity
DIOXINS	Released into the air from burning materials, diesel fuel, petroleum, etc. They are in the air and end up in water and	All cancers Immune system dysfunction Reproductive system dysfunction	Lowers sperm count later in life due to intrauterine exposure in boys

	animal products		
PCBs	Industrial coolants & lubricants	Skin cancer Liver cancer Brain cancer Disrupts thyroid hormone Disrupts liver function Contributes to diabetes	Increases childhood obesity when exposed in the womb
PHTHAL- ATES	Plastic food containers Children’s toys PVC Plastic wrap with #3 label Personal care products labeled “fragrance” Air fresheners	Causes cell death in testicles Lower sperm count Lower sperm motility Obesity Diabetes Thyroid dys- regulation	Birth defects in male reproductive system Also disrupts the masculine neurological development when exposed in the womb
PERCHLO- RATE	Jet fuel that affects: Produce Milk Tap water	Competes with iodine and causes thyroid dysfunction	May alter brain development and organ development

	**Drink filtered water		in the fetus, infants and young children
FIRE RETARDANTS (Poly-brominated diphenyl esthers)	Found every-where in industry produced products—couches, carpet, clothing, etc. **Use HEPA filter with your vacuum **Avoid re-upholstering furniture **Avoid carpet foam	Thyroid dys-regulation	Thyroid disruption Alters brain development Learning disabilities Lowers IQ
XENO-ESTROGENS	Plastics Additional release if plastics are heated. **Never microwave plastic Tap water Styrofoam	Disrupts normal hormone metabolism & can cause infertility Also, contributes to estrogen based cancers	Affects developing sex organs and may cause defects

		(breast, ovary, etc)	
LEAD	Old paint Drinking water Older children's toys	Miscarriage Kidney damage Nervous system damage Hormone disruption High blood pressure Diabetes Anxiety De-pression	Brain damage Lowered IQ Hearing loss Fetal death Premature birth
ARSENIC	Water Some wood stains such as picnic tables and play structures	Skin cancer Lung cancer Bladder cancer Interferes with normal hormone and how it processes sugar & carbo-hydrates thus weight problems, protein wasting,	Low birth weight Fetal Loss Possible de-velopmental delays

		immune suppression, insulin resistance, osteoporosis, growth retardation and high blood pressure	
MERCURY	Certain seafood, sushi in particular	Binds to certain hormones which regulate menstrual cycles & ovulation Diabetes Pancreatic damage Insulin disruption	Concentrates in the fetal brain and causes brain damage
PFC'S (Perfluo-rinated chemi-cals)	Non-stick cookware Stain resistant carpet Carpet cleaning	Decreases sperm quality Interferes with hormone production	Low birth weight Early breast development Delayed puberty

	agents Microwave popcorn	Kidney disease & cancer Testicular cancer Thyroid disease Elevated cholesterol May also be linked to Ulcerative colitis Pre-eclampsia	
ORGAN-OPHOS-PHATE PESTI-CIDES	Pesticides	Affects the nervous system Contributes to infertility Affects testosterone levels Alters thyroid levels	Affects brain development, the nervous system & causes behavioral issues
GLYCOL ETHERS	Paint solvents Household Cleaning products	Causes testicular shrinkage Lower's sperm count	Can cause permanent damage to the fetus' reproductive

	Brake fluid Cosmetics		organs Childhood asthma Childhood allergies

(DIRTY DOZEN ENDOCRINE DISRUPTORS, n.d.)

(National Institute of Environmental Health Sciences, n.d.)

(Xenoestrogens, n.d.) (Fahmida Tofail, 2009)

PLASTICS

Plastics emit xenoestrogens, especially when heated. Xenoestrogens are endocrine disruptors that can interfere with fertility in both men and women. They are attributed to miscarriages and hormonal conditions such as endometriosis and early onset puberty. Xenoestrogens have also been linked to hormonal cancers such as prostate and breast cancer, obesity, testicular cancer, and diabetes. Xenoestrogens are listed individually above but they are really part of several of the chemicals discussed in this book such as phthalates, BPA, pesticides, herbicides, PCBs et cetera. I wanted to add a section here to discuss the use of plastics for food and water. One simple thing you can do is try to get rid of most of your plastics you have for storing food. There are several companies out there that make glass based containers; the lids will be plastic but that isn't as bad because it is not in contact with the food. Never, ever heat food in a plastic container, even if it says BPA free. Avoid using plastic wrap to store or heat food. If you have a plastic water botte that has been in your hot car or has been heated in any capacity, throw it away. In fact, try to do away with plastic water bottles as much as possible. There are several glass and stainless steel brands and options available for purchase that you can fill up and carry with you wherever you go. In all honesty, water will likely still come from plastic at some point but decreasing your exposure definitely helps. Simply put, control what you can, when you can to minimize damage to yourself and your baby.

(LaRue, 2012) (A List of Xenoestrogens, 2014) (Xenohormones and Xenoestrogens)

CHAPTER 7

DIETARY CONSIDERATIONS

People will often choose to stick their head in the sand when it comes to diet because people don't like to change what they know and do and have done for their whole life, especially when it comes to food. Unfortunately, when it comes to food, it can have a huge impact on your overall health and ultimately, your ability to conceive. Every new patient I have receives a folder which includes several handouts, including one called "Basic Food Tips". I am going to review the contents of that handout plus add a few details in relation to fertility.

1. Choose whole foods or "foods of the earth". If you can pick it and eat it or hunt it/pick it, cook it and eat it, your body knows what to do with it, otherwise, avoid it.
    - To aid in choosing a whole foods diet, do "perimeter shopping". The perimeter of the grocery store is where you find the fresh foods, everything in between is the processed garbage.
    - Meat is fine in its purest form, limit deli meats or prepared meats. There are some deli meats that do not have added chemicals (nitrates/nitrites) in them that can be used for lunch meat.

- When it comes to dairy, milk is ok but yogurt is better. ALWAYS choose organic whenever available; it is worth the extra dollar!
- Buy organic, plain, nonfat yogurt and add the fruit yourself; it's higher in protein and lower in sugars. Try adding just cinnamon for even less sugar!
- Use cheese sparingly and never use processed cheese like Velveeta or individually wrapped cheese slices. Key words to avoid are: "processed cheese product" in the ingredient list.
- Soymilk is processed and often the crops are heavily dosed with pesticides as well as genetically modified. In some cases, organic soy milk may be a better alternative to cow's milk but almond or coconut milk would be a better first choice. In these cases, choose organic whenever possible.
- Margarine is NOT food and is packed full of added chemicals which are toxic to your body. The ingredients in butter? "Cream and salt" ...it doesn't get much simpler than that! ALWAYS choose organic if possible.
- "Instant—anything" is processed and stripped of fiber. There are some exceptions to this—organic instant oatmeal retains its fiber. Try to stick with plain to keep sugar consumption lower. You can add your own fruit and nuts.
- Juice and juicing is not typically recommended. Juicing takes the sugary part and leaves the fiber behind. Wouldn't you rather eat two apples or

oranges than drink 8 ounces of juice? Plus, pure juice is hard to come by and expensive! If you want to make a "juice", I recommend using a Blender, Bullet, VitaMix or something similar. This allows you to use the whole fruit or whole vegetable in the machine and preserve the "wholeness" of the produce.

2. Avoid or limit "white food" such as white rice, white bread, pasta, and potatoes. Choose "100% whole wheat breads" or "sprouted wheat". Choose quinoa, brown rice, and if you must have a pasta, use quinoa or whole-wheat pasta. Use yams or sweet potatoes instead of potatoes as these have more nutrients and fiber.

3. Avoid "diet" foods or foods labeled at "lite/light" as these contain synthetic sugars such as aspartame, known to cause cancer and many chronic diseases. Low fat and non-fat is ok in most instances but check labels.

4. Avoid *trans*-fats! Your body does not know what to do with these adulterated fats and will accumulate in your vessels. Look for the word "hydrogenated" on labels if buying processed foods. The process of hydrogenation turns naturally occurring, *cis*-configuration of fats into a *trans*-configuration of fats. The purpose is to increase shelf life and change melting points. If it has been hydrogenated, it has *trans*-fats so don't believe the

claims that it doesn't! They may have decreased but they are still there.

5. Buy Organic whenever possible. Yes, it is more expensive most of the time but it's your body and food is nourishment!

6. Always choose fresh or frozen vegetables or fruit. It is best to almost NEVER chose canned. Some exceptions may be things such as artichoke hearts and olives but both of these can be found in jars as well and is preferable. If you do use cans, looks for those with liners labeled as "BPA free" especially in acidic foods such as tomato.

7. Your refrigerator should be loaded and your pantry relatively sparse. This indicates a primarily whole foods diet. In the pantry should be bulk grains and foods.

8. Buy mason or canning jars to put your bulk grains in for easier access and more appeal.

9. Water should be bottled or filtered, even for cooking. Try a Brita or Pur filtration system attached to your faucet. They are relatively inexpensive and easy to use.

10. Make your grocery shopping experience fun and never rushed. Plan at least 2 hours to get to the store, spend

time looking (especially if you are seeing "the perimeter" for the first time!"), then go home and prepare for the week.

11. Preparation for the week means that you don't unload your groceries feeling like you have accomplished something by going shopping because there is more to it than that. Now you have to make the food accessible so you can be successful.
    - Chop veggies, make a veggie tray with hummus dip for quick snacks,
    - Wash fruits and make an "easy access fruit bowl" for quick grabs.
    - Chop lettuce and salad toppings for quick salad preparation during the busy times.
    - Bake chicken breasts or fish then dice to add protein to salads.
    - This whole process can take time so budget it into your schedule and save time later!

12. Sample lunch/dinner plate:
    - Split your plate in fourths either literally or mentally.
        - ❑ Fresh veggies—provides enzymes and fiber specific to fresh.
        - ❑ Cooked/steamed—balances the body and aids in digestion
        - ❑ Protein—choose lean meats and deep-water fish. If you are a vegetarian or want a break from meat, choose tofu or

meat-alternatives. You may also substitute beans here on occasion.

- Carbohydrate—this area includes all grains, legumes (beans, peas, etc) and starchy vegetables.
    - Grains: brown rice, quinoa, kamut, millet, oats, whole wheat, amaranth, spelt, buckwheat, etc.
    - Legumes: beans (black beans, kidney beans, garbanzo beans green beans, etc), peas, lentils, etc.
    - Starchy vegetables: corn, yams, sweet potatoes, etc.

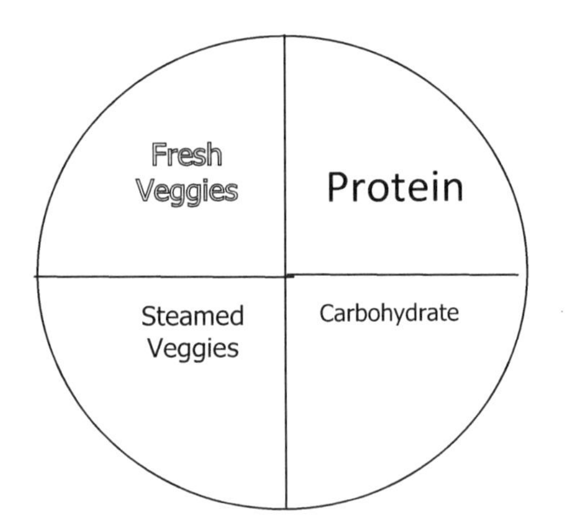

I suppose I could stop there and hope that you follow the recommendations to a T but I want to elaborate on some of the basic points made above and how the things I recommend you avoid can be detrimental to your health.

DELI MEATS & OTHER PROCESSED MEATS

As you may know, deli meats have the potential to cause Listeria in pregnant women and this may cause death of the baby. It is recommended that all deli meats be cooked if you choose to eat them but it is ideal to avoid them altogether to be on the safe side. Listeria is a serious problem when it comes to deli meat and still kills about 500 people per year with a 20% fatality rate.

Although Listeria is frightening, this is NOT the reason I am discussing deli meats. The other problem with deli meats goes well beyond the days of pregnancy. This information is for you, your spouse and your current and future children. The problem with most deli meats is that if it doesn't say "nitrate free" then there are nitrates in it. Check the label and you will see for yourself. Nitrates in particular are extremely harmful to you and also to your developing baby and once baby is born, should continue to be kept out of baby's diet on a regular basis.

Processed meats include: bacon, sausage, ham, jerky, deli turkey, deli ham, deli chicken, all regular cold cuts, salami, pepperoni, hot dogs, bratwurst, breakfast links & patties, et cetera.

I have known there is a risk and correlation to cancer when it comes to nitrates for over a decade but recent research finally landed into the mainstream media in the last couple of years. The American Institute for cancer research reports that 3.5 ounces of processed meat per day (the amount in a typical sandwich) increases your risk of colorectal cancer by 36%. In 2012, CBC news reported on a study publish in the British Journal of Cancer that showed a 19% increase in pancreatic cancer with a daily serving of processed meat. And in 2006, the TODAY Show educated that nitrates are converted to nitrites which bind to DNA and are associated with cancer of the mouth, bladder, stomach, brain and esophagus. They also reported Swedish studies that showed one serving per day increased stomach cancer by 15%.

NCBI published an article in Environmental Health Journal that reported nitrites can be found in the public water supply and may be harmful to pregnant women and unborn fetuses so if you choose to avoid deli meat, its best to close the loop by drinking filtered water whenever possible. This was revisited later in the journal Environmental Health Perspectives and published on the Environmental Health News website where they reported nitrites in water were definitively linked to cleft palate, limb deformities, heart defects and spina bifida. Of note, these studies were done in Texas and Iowa due to heavy pesticide & fertilizer use in the area that infiltrates the local drinking water and aquifers.

With all that being said, these risks go beyond your own health. As the free radicals and cancer-causing agents pulse through you, they also go to your baby and can affect him/her in the same way. Perhaps this is a link and correlation as to why we have a rise in childhood cancers. They always seem like such a mystery but perhaps they are not so mysterious after all. In fact, the FDA has put sodium nitrite in the drug category C which if you reference previous material, you will see it is a KNOWN fact that it causes damage and death in fetuses, both human and animal. In addition, Public Health Nutrition published a study that stated there is a link to brain cancer in babies of mother's who consumed cured (deli) meat on a regular basis.

Knowledge is power and in the case of health, that power can aid in prevention.

(TODAY: 5 things you need to know about deli meats, 2006)

(FAQ: Processed Meats and Cancer, 2014)

(Bacon, deli meat may raise pancreatic cancer risk, 2012)

(Deana M Manassaram, 2010)

(Sodium Nitrate Consumption During Pregnancy, 2015)

(Sodium nitrite / sodium thiosulfate Pregnancy and Breastfeeding Warnings, n.d.)

(JD Brender, 2013)

(The Dangers of Nitrites: The Foods They are Found In and Why You Want to Avoid Them, n.d.)

SOY MILK & OTHER SOY PRODUCTS

Soy milk has long been touted as a "health food" and alternative to milk. Mention the word "tofu" to most people and they automatically cringe and think you are going to take away their hamburger. Soy beans were originally brought to the US as livestock feed in the form of plants and were then used to create plastics and oils in the automobile industry. After World War 2, soybean meal was added to livestock feed allowing mass production of livestock for consumption. Ben Franklin introduced America to soy as a food as tofu and over the years, it has infiltrated our food supply as a health food, a vegetarian alternative to meat and as a bulking agent in processed foods including fast food hamburgers.

The main concern with soy in relation to your future baby is that it does have estrogenic properties. Soy contains "phytoestrogens" which, in an adult female, may be helpful in cases of low estrogen but harmful in cases of high estrogen as the phytoestrogens compete for binding sites on the estrogen receptors. What that means is that if you don't have enough estrogen, phytoestrogens can increase estrogens on the tissues that need it (a good thing in moderation). If you have too much estrogen, phytoestrogens can decrease the overall estrogenic effect on the tissues that have estrogen receptors. In the case of someone who has normal estrogen, soy can interfere by either increasing estrogen effects at the receptors or decreasing natural estrogen effects by binding in place of natural estrogen. As it applies for the babies: if you have a baby girl in your womb, she will get excess estrogen too early for her body; if you have a boy, he will get way too much estrogen than he will ever need and at a vulnerable time.

There may be some correlation to birth defects such as hypospadias (a condition where the opening to the urethra develops on the bottom side of the penis) and cryptorchidism (absence of one or both testes in the scrotum) in boys and some studies have found that women who ate a soy-focused vegetarian diet had nearly 5 times greater risk of having a boy born with hypospadias. Research also shows that masculinization may be affected in prenatal exposure to phytoestrogens and that consumption by males during puberty may result in a smaller penis size and feminization of male genitals.

It is also speculated by many, and in my opinion, cannot be ruled out, that phytoestrogens will produce the same or similar outcomes as xenoestrogens such as predisposition to estrogen receptive cancers as well as possibly contribute to struggles with fertility. For men who consume excessive phytoestrogens, the artificially elevated estrogens can cause low sperm count, low motility, poor sperm quality and decreased libido. The conclusion here is simple, limit soy in your diet if you are trying to get pregnant or are already pregnant. Limit soy if you are male or a child.

(History of Soybeans, n.d.)

(Soy Foods Are Part of America's History, n.d.)

(Daniels, n.d.) (Carmichael SL1 & Study, 2013, Aug 1) (SoyOnline Service, n.d.)

(Vegetarian Diets and Birth Defects, 2000) (Poggi, 2005)

GENTICALLY MODIFIED FOODS

GMO foods or Genetically Modified Organisms are plants whose DNA has been altered by science to benefit the plant's production or shelf-life. Scientists use bacteria or viruses to incorporate various things or "options" into the genetic make-up of the plant. It can make it resistant to herbicides and pesticides, make it grow bigger, keep it from bruising, keep it from turning brown once cut and other seemingly good benefits. This allows more produce to be created at a faster speed and at less loss to the farmers. In addition, it makes the foods more appealing on the grocery shelves by appearing more radiant in color, flawless, bigger, juicier, etc. The problem is that we don't know the long-term effects and as we have more people becoming chronically ill "no reason" there may be a finger to point after all. Medicine has developed more "syndromes" over the years because people are sick and we don't know why…but maybe we do actually know. We can't change the way people eat because everyone is addicted to convenience. Its speculated that at least 80% of processed food in the United States is genetically modified. If it doesn't say non-GMO then it probably falls into that category.

Some of the most genetically modified crops are corn (85%) and soy (91%) and cotton (88%). Other common crops include: rapeseed, canola, honey, rice, sugar, tomatoes, sweet corn, potatoes, flax, papaya, squash, peas, sugar beets and vegetable oils.

How does this affect your health and the health of your baby? If you put GMO soy into a search engine, one of the first articles that comes up is the link between GMO soy, sterility and infant mortality. A recent study on goats in Italy showed that growth was slowed by 20% in baby goats whose mothers were fed GMO soy because it altered the composition of their breast-milk by lowering fat and protein. The milk had lowered IgG antibodies present thus making the baby goats more susceptible to infection and underdeveloped gut function (one of the primary responsibilities of the IgG). It is also known that GMO soy has a "residue" that can be found in blood after consumption. That "residue" is called glyphosate and has been linked to various cancers, particularly of the reproductive tract. It also causes growth and development disruptions in offspring. In addition, studies report that it may cause deformities of the brain, heart and intestines plus infertility, miscarriages, sterility and endocrine dysfunction. The bottom line is that genetically modified foods can and will affect your health on a long-term basis and will undoubtedly affect your baby both currently and in his or her future, we just don't know the full extent as of yet.

(Genetically Modified Foods, n.d.)

(Amy Paturel and Robin Yamakawa Reviewed by Brunilda Nazario, 2015)

(Langtree, 2009) (Jonathan Latham, 2015) (Gutierrez, 2015)

(Glyphosate: The Toxin So Dangerous, It's Causing Catastrophic Birth Defects, 2012)

DAIRY

I often get a little anxious when I talk about dairy, mostly because people love their dairy and they get VERY defensive about it when I bring it up, even if it is the primary cause of all their discomfort and poor health. As children grow up they are inundated by the media, government, schools, parents, et cetera who all touted dairy as the end all, be all, dietary requirement for proper growth and nutrition. Right? In 2013, I spent a day at a local high school discussing basic nutrition and supplements to teens. In the last section of the day, when I mentioned that dairy can actually leach calcium out of bones, there was a full-on uproar as if I told them they were all adopted. It was so shocking and somewhat amusing to witness their reaction to this information as I essentially told them they have been lied to since birth. I also want to add, as many of the supporters of the anti-dairy move do, that we were not designed to be dependent on cattle for our survival or nutrition. People get "grossed out" about breast milk or breast feeding in public, while sipping their latte which came from the breasts of COWS! I am not sure how we got so turned around in our thinking but we have, and we are, and we need to work toward change. We are the only mammals on the planet that continue to consume milk after we are weaned. We are all stuck in the habit of suckling the milk nectar long after our bodies are in need of the nutrient dense substance, which I might add, is designed for building fat and muscle for baby cows which have to quickly support their growing one-ton bodies. It was not designed for our human babies who are tiny in comparison and need brain food, not muscle food. It certainly was NOT designed for adult humans who do not need any encouragement in the "growth" department most of the time.

That being said, here are some shocking facts about milk/dairy:

1. It leaches calcium from bones.
2. The proteins are huge and are designed for baby cows which have 4 stomachs. Humans have one

stomach so the large proteins are impossible for us to break down properly.

3. Dairy promotes inflammation which can exacerbate or contribute to nearly any disease including heart disease, autoimmune disease, asthma, allergies, eczema, etc.
4. Dairy has been definitively linked to Type 1 (child-onset) diabetes by damaging the pancreas, especially if introduced too early in life.
5. Non-organic milk (specifically milk with rBGH—a hormone given to cows to increase milk production) is linked to several cancers including breast and prostate cancer.

The most profoundly shocking article I came across in my research comes from Physicians Committee of Responsible Medicine. They reported the following shocking statistics:

1. Daily consumption of 3 or more glasses of milk per day (24 ounces – equivalent to two tall lattes!) showed:
    a. A 60% higher rate of hip fracture later in life.
    b. A 93% higher mortality rate.
2. Risk of dying from all illnesses increases by 15% for every 8-ounce glass of milk consumed on a daily basis.
3. Without adequate Vitamin D, calcium is not properly absorbed, in fact, only 10-15% of calcium can be absorbed if you are Vitamin D deficient.

4. Dairy intake is associated with heart disease due to its high fat content.
5. Dairy is the leading contributor to dioxin intake in our diet. (reference the Environmental Toxins chart above—dioxins cause cancer and also low sperm count)

If the facts and statistic here are not enough, I encourage you to do your own research online. There are many, many articles, both opinion and research based that will support everything written here. Dairy is loved by all but it is damaging your body on a daily basis. Consider eliminating it completely or at minimum, reducing your consumption.

(Osteoporosis Milk Myth, n.d.) (Health Concerns about Dairy Products, n.d.)

(Dairy & It's Effects on Health, 2011) (Brookover, n.d.)

PROCESSED CHEESE

Most of this section can be summarized by reading the preceding sections on dairy and environmental toxins and the sections following this on processed foods and additives but I want to use this opportunity to educate you on what processed cheese actually is. As the name implies, it is "processed" and usually contains very little cheese at all. As Americans, we tend to favor processed foods in general, which is likely why we have gifted it the name of "American Cheese", when it comes to those lovely cheese slices that appear on most fast food burgers around the country. Although originally created by a Swiss scientist, it was patented by an American and went live with Kraft Company here in the United States. Processed cheese is created by taking a small amount of dairy and adding colors, preservatives and flavors as well as binders, fillers, and additives. The economic benefit is that it is less expensive to make so it is cheaper on the shelf, it can last weeks, months or even years outside the refrigerator and it is made in perfect shapes that match typical white bread loaves for perfect sandwiches and of course, it melts faster at lower temperatures for those all-American burgers or nachos. Interesting to note, that cheese slices won't melt at high temperatures and rather takes on a plastic-like appearance if placed in an open flame (I encourage you to watch a video on this!). Processed cheese is packed full of toxic chemicals, most of which land on the top worst food additive's chart (see below).

(What is Processed Cheese, n.d.) (What's in processed cheese slices?, 2015)

PROCESSED FOODS: ADDITIVES, COLORING AGENTS, ARTIFICIAL SWEETENERS & MORE

In addition to the content already covered, I want to take a moment to promote a whole foods diet once again by highlighting all the negative aspects of the toxic chemicals added to food in order to make them shelf-stable, able to be packaged, addictive to the palate for repeat purchase and consumption, appealing to the eye, et cetera. We live in a world of convenience and it is coming at a price. Our epidemic of disease is spreading and most of the top diseases can somehow be tied back to our reliance on convenience foods. Obviously, this book is on what to do during pre-conception, during pregnancy and the first year after. So, if cutting out processed foods seems like something you absolutely cannot do for yourself, do it for your baby during this precious time. You are obviously willing to make that sacrifice or you would not be taking the time to read this material. Your baby's exposure to these chemicals can be exponential compared to yours when he or she is in the womb. In my research, I read an article from a mother than is fairly certain her son is mentally handicapped due to her consumption of aspartame and phenylalanine supplements while she was pregnant. She now has to live with that for the rest of her life. So just as you would not consume alcohol or smoke cigarettes, put these processed foods in the same category for this period of time and ideally, limit your child's exposure in the first few years of life.

(The Aspartame Controversy, n.d.)

Here is a chart to guide you regarding Processed Food Additives, why they add them to food, what foods they add them to and what diseases they are associated with:

ADDITIVE	PURPOSE	LOCATION	DISEASES or PROBLEMS THEY CAUSE
Propyl Gallate	Preservative; prevents spoiling of fats	Chewing gum Chicken stock Potato sticks Meat products Vegetable oil	Cancer
BHA/BHT	Preservative	Gum Cereal Vegetable oil Potato chips	Endocrine Disruptor Infertility Cancer
Potassium Bromate	Increases volume and help make the flour finer and crumbly	Breads	Cancer
Monosodium glutamate (MSG)	Flavor enhancer	Soup Salad dressing Sausage & hot dogs Canned tuna Potato	Produces "excitotoxins" which can cause brain tissue to die.

		chips Candy	
High Fructose Corn Syrup	Sweetener	Candy Baked goods Crackers Most packaged foods	Mitochondrial malfunction Obesity
Aspartame	Artificial sweetener (Nutra-Sweet & Equal)	Diet sodas “Light” foods & “Diet” foods Chewing gum	Brain tumors Lymphoma Leukemia Birth defects (physical such as eye placement and neural tube defects such as spina bifida) Affects brain development in unborn fetuses
Sucralose / Splenda	Artificial Sweetener	Diet sodas “Light” foods & “Diet” foods Chewing gum	Inflammatory Bowel Disease Inactivates digestive enzymes Damages the normal gut barrier Kills normal

			gut flora
Acesulfame-K	Artificial sweetener	Baked goods Gum Gelatin desserts (such as Jell-O) Soft Drinks	Thyroid disease May alter neurologic function
Olestra	Fat substitute	Crackers & chips labeled as Fat Free or Low Fat	Decreased nutrient absorption
Diacetyl	Butter flavoring	Microwave popcorn	Alzheimer's disease
Sodium Nitrite/ Nitrate	Preservative & flavoring	Processed meats	Cancer, particularly colon, stomach and pancreatic
Sodium Benzoate & Potassium Benzoate	Mold preventative	Soda/soft drinks	Cancer Thyroid damage and disease Hyperactivity
Hydrogenated Vegetable Oil "Trans Fats"	Fat preservative	Margarine Vegetable shortening Crackers Cookies Baked goods Salad	May cause cancer by deactivation of our natural cancer fighting enzymes Interfere with insulin

		dressings Breads	receptors and cause diabetes Decrease immune system Infertility—they damage enzymes needed to manufacture hormones May cause heart disease
Blue 1 & 2	Color additive	Beverages Baked goods Candy	Cancer Brain tumors
Red 3	Color additive	Cherries such as maraschino & fruit cocktail Baked goods Candy	Thyroid tumors Cancer—various Allergies Hyperactivity Aggression Learning impairment
Red 40	Color additive	Candy Baked goods Cereal Beverages	Immune system tumors Cancer—various Allergies Hyperactivity Aggression

			Learning impairment
Yellow 5	Color additive	Candy Baked goods Cereal Beverages	Cancer—various types Allergies Hyperactivity Hyper-sensitivity Behavioral changes Learning impairment
Yellow 6	Color additive	Baked goods Candy Gelatin Sausages	Adrenal tumors Kidney tumors Carcinogenic and may cause other cancers Allergies Hyperactivity Aggression Learning impairment

(Dirty Dozen Food Additives, n.d.) (Michaels, 2013) (Mercola, 2013) (Evans, 2010) (Milton Stokes, 2010) (Curran, 2010)

In addition to the chemicals that are actually added to food in the processing, there are also toxic chemicals in the packaging material themselves. This makes sense as boxes and bags don't grow naturally in nature, they have to be created and most of them have some sort of plastic involved. Some of the chemicals used include:

1. Formaldehyde in soda bottles to prevent mold, which is linked to cancer and autoimmune diseases.
2. Melamine in plastic food containers & utensils which is linked to kidney stones, kidney failure and kidney cancer (in 2008, 50,000 babies became ill and 3 ultimately died from melamine in formula containers)
3. BPA in canned food liners (discussed above) and is an endocrine disruptor and also linked to obesity, asthma, behavioral issues, kidney & heart disease. **In this same family: tributyltin, triclosan, phthalates
4. Phthalates are located in plastic containers for toys and food containers. They are linked to premature birth and insulin resistance (type 2 diabetes)

There comes a point that you have to be realistic though and although these things exist, they are essentially unavoidable unless you grow your own food. You can take action to limit your exposure (for example, Amy's Organic Soups now uses BPA free cans) but try to be reasonable because if it is too overwhelming, you might give up altogether. The goal again is to LIMIT what goes into your body. As I have stated multiple times, we are talking about the two-year window for your baby. Most people can do anything if they know it is not forever and this is what I am encouraging you to do.

(Graham, 2014)

TRANS-FATS

A short note on Trans-Fats—I briefly covered it in the chart above as a food additive but it is also a stand-alone ingredient with its own winning or rather, not-so-winning personality. Trans-fats are created by taking a regular fat/oil and adding a hydrogen in order to turn a liquid fat into a solid fat in order to add flavor, texture, prolong shelf life and lower production costs to processed foods. These types of adulterated fats are a common ingredient in processed foods, mostly under the name of "partially-hydrogenated fats/oils", now commonly referred to as PFO's. They are found in pie crusts, ready to eat frosting, biscuits, cookies, baked goods, crackers, doughnuts, various chips and related snack foods, coffee creamer, margarine, and almost all fried foods. You may have it in your house as shortening as well so this is a good time to check and if you have it, get rid of it.

It has been found that these fats increase your bad cholesterol (LDL), lower your good cholesterol (HDL) and ultimately put you at risk for heart disease and stroke. They also have been associated with memory loss, an increase in inflammation, insulin resistance, obesity and type 2 diabetes.

As recently as June of 2015, the FDA has made a move to require all food manufacturing companies to remove trans-fats from their ingredients as they have finally deemed it unsafe for human consumption. Medical experts feel that if this decision is implemented, there will be a palpable decrease in cardiovascular disease in the years to come (up to 250,000 less deaths per year).

The obvious next question is whether or not consumption of trans-fats can affect your baby while in the womb or during breast feeding. There is evidence published by the American Journal of Clinical Nutrition that showed increase in birth weight in babies whose mother consumed a diet rich in trans-fats. Additional research found that after birth, growth was slowed and glucose sensitivity was affected. It is speculated that mother's consumption of trans-fats may predispose children to obesity and diabetes later in life but research is still underway for these hypotheses.

(Skarnulis, 2014)

(Trans Fats is double trouble for your heart health, 2015)

(AHA: Trans Fats, 2015) (FDA: Trans Fats, 2015) (Christensen, 2015)

(Eating More Trans Fats Could Be Bad for Memory, 2015)

(The Nutrition Source: Shining the Spot Light on TransFats, n.d.)

(Juliana FW Cohen, 2011, Nov) (K, et al., 2010) (Thomas, 2011)

In conclusion for this chapter on nutrition, I am sure many people are feeling a bit overwhelmed. I want to reference you back to the start of the chapter regarding Basic Food Tips as there are examples of what a "whole foods diet" looks like. Basically, it comes down to vegetables, fruits, lean meats and whole grains. There are many resources out there to help guide you so that you don't go to extremes. And yet another reminder that the focus of this book is on the two years you are devoting to your baby and his/her future health on all aspects: physical, mental and emotional in order to give them the best chance at being as "perfect" as you can make them.

CHAPTER 8

EXERCISE

Exercise is a topic that is about as much fun to bring up to patients as cutting out dairy. The bottom line is that most people do not enjoy exercise. If you do, you are an exception to the rule. People also don't like hard work and they don't like to do things that they don't find "fun". I have heard countless excuses as to why people don't exercise. Most people don't have time (although they have plenty of time to watch TV at night) and a big portion don't like to go to the gym because it is "boring" which always makes me chuckle a little as I wonder if I am speaking to a grown up or if my 7-year old is sitting in front of me. I tell everyone that when it comes to things like exercise, we have to parent our inner child. That may sound "weird" but here is what I mean—we all have an internal battle, right? So, when your inner voices, says (with a child-like tone) "I don't want to, I am too tired, it's boring, I will do it tomorrow, do I HAVE to?" You have to sternly say to yourself that you have to exercise, it's a priority and it's important to your health. Exercise should be as important as sleep and food on a regular basis. I have started pointing out to my patients that if you put those 3 things in the same category, you will be more successful. You would not skip sleeping because you are too busy and if you did, it would not be for more than one day. You would not skip eating due to being too busy and if you did, it would not be for more than a meal or two. Treat exercise the same way you would eating and sleeping and make it a "non-negotiable" in your daily life. If you have to skip it, don't do it for more than a day or two before forcing yourself to get back on track.

EXERCISE VS. FITNESS

Exercise is intentional movement for the purpose of improved health and prevention of illness while "fitness" is defined more as a measure of your ability to perform daily functions with adequate energy and vigor. Fitness is relative and variable and there is no clear indication at which time you personally have achieved ultimate "fitness" but regular exercise is the only way to get there.

Physical Fitness requires 3 components:

Cardiorespiratory Endurance

This is the sustained ability of "the system" to carry oxygen to your cells. Cardiorespiratory endurance is obtained with "aerobic" activities such as brisk walking, running, cycling, etc.

Muscular Fitness

This is the ability of your muscles to lift and pull at least your own weight and the ability to perform repeated contractions in quick succession.

Flexibility
The ability to move your body and limbs in their full range of motion without discomfort.

TOP BENEFITS OF EXERCISE

There are many benefits to exercise and we all know them or get the gist of them but here they are laid out for you to remind yourself why you need to just do it anyway, even when you don't want to. These benefits are for general health of course. In the next section, we will discuss benefits to you in relation to pregnancy and your baby.

1. Exercise strengthens your heart and lungs; a.k.a. the cardiovascular and respiratory systems
    a. Exercise lowers the buildup of plaques in the arteries by increasing your "good" cholesterol and decreasing the "bad" cholesterol in the blood. These plaques are what increase your blood pressure over time as they build up so the overall effect is twofold! It lowers cholesterol AND blood pressure!
    b. Exercise promotes rhythmic and deep breathing and increases the overall capacity of the lungs. Larger lung capacity means more space for oxygen exchange and more oxygen means providing better nourishment to cells which means better cellular metabolism! It also increases circulation

keeping you warmer in cooler weather and cooler in warmer weather. Isn't the body amazing!?!?

   c. Because you have a stronger heart and lungs and more oxygen is getting to your tissues, this also means more energy and better sleep.

2. Keeps bones and muscles strong
   a. "Impact" or weight bearing exercises causes a release of "bone building armies" called osteoblasts. They strengthen your bones and decrease your risk of developing osteoporosis.
   b. Strong muscles have an effect on bones because they provide a constant pull on the bones they attach to which also decreases your risk of osteoporosis.
   c. Another factor is that increasing strength usually means increasing balance and coordination decreasing the risk of falls and ultimately fractures.
3. Weight management
   a. Burning more calories will help you lose weight. Even after your done with our workout, your body continues to burn more calories for the next few hours. By exercising with a healthy diet, you are burning more calories than you take in, you reduce body fat and increase lean body mass thus lowering your overall BMI and decreasing your risk for obesity.

   b. By managing weight, you also decrease risk for heart disease, diabetes, arthritis, cancer and many other diseases.

4. Prevents (and manages) diabetes
   a. Exercise helps your insulin to work better and can lower your blood sugar because your muscles are using up sugars for fuel/energy to work more efficiently. And remember this process continues for hours after your workout. Seems like diabetics would benefit from several brisk walks a day…don't you think?
   b. Exercise also increases your cellular sensitivity to insulin so your body can use it more efficiently to bring energy (sugar) into your cells.
5. Eases depression; manages stress; decrease pain
   a. Exercise causes an increase in neurotransmitters—the little chemicals that make us happy or help us deal with stress or pain.
      - Serotonin gives us feelings of wellbeing and staves off depression.
      - Norepinephrine balances stress hormones and anxiety.
      - Endorphins such as GABA provide pain relief as well as relaxation.
6. Finding the energy to go after work can change your life. Instead of going for an addictive substance (alcohol, food, television) after a hard day, allow your body to do its own work! Take a brisk 30-

minute walk and then sit back and enjoy the side effects!

7. Improves learning and memory and prevents cognitive decline.
    a. Studies show that just 10 minutes of vigorous exercise can improve scores on task that require extra attention. In addition, studies show that even mild exercise can maintain memory and cognitive function as we age.
    b. Also, even if genetically predisposed to Alzheimer's disease, people who worked out regularly were significantly less likely to express the genes that cause Alzheimer's.
8. Improves self-esteem
    a. Studies show that achieving your own fitness goals or improving your fitness level helps boost self-esteem and of course, by nature, your body image will improve as an added bonus.
9. Improves libido and sexual function
    a. Exercise decreases incidence of erectile function in men.
    b. It has been shown to improve sexual arousal in women.
10. Improves sleep
    a. Due to the release of the neurotransmitters, your tissues getting more oxygen and your body needing more rest and repair time in general, a good work out can improve your sleep dramatically.

    b. Try to do your cardio at least 3 hours before bedtime, as the initial response is a surge in energy for some people (although not the case for everyone).
11. Reduces risk of some cancers
    a. Exercise has been linked to a lower risk of hormonally related cancers such as breast, prostate, colon and uterine cancers.
    b. With colon cancer, it is speculated that exercise improves digestion overall thus lowering the risk of harmful substances staying in the colon and causing damage.
    c. Uterine and breast cancer risk is decreased by decreasing overall body fat and decreasing estrogen production (peripheral conversion).
    d. Prostate cancer risk is lowered because...well, we are still unsure but more than likely it is due to an improvement in overall hormonal balancing.
12. Improves longevity and quality of life
    a. Over time, as the body ages, tasks become more difficult. The more in shape you are, the less likely this will happen.
    b. You will live longer due to the overall improvement in health.
    c. Studies show that you have a 40% less chance of early death with 7 hours per week of exercise.
    d. Your longer life will be fuller because you will be able to do more things than the average 80-90-year-old!

(Sarnataro, n.d.) (Physical Activity and Health, n.d.) (Deborah Kotz, 2012)

(Exercise: 7 benefits of regular physical activity, 2014)

REQUIREMENTS

Yes, I said requirements, not recommendations. Obviously, no one can MAKE you do anything but the government has even called these "requirements". It is the minimum amount required to prevent disease and maintain health. So, they aren't really recommendations because the general medical field and the government wants people to stay healthy as it costs billions of dollars per year to pay for the people who view it as only a "recommendation" and therefore become ill due to lack of activity. Sedentary has become the norm but we are genetically programmed to work to survive and we just don't do it anymore. Due to the lack of necessary "work" just to survive, we now have to go to the gym or brave the elements to achieve a level of fitness that our body requires to sustain health.

For adults, the CDC and American Heart Association both recommend 150 minutes per week of moderate activity or 75 minutes of vigorous activity plus 2 days a week of some sort of weight training for adults. The general rule is 30 minutes 5 days a week, however, this amount increases for weight loss and disease control (meaning you already have an issue and you are trying to fix it). The World Health Organization recommends double the amount listed here for *optimal* health. Basically, if you have not done the minimum most of your life, you now have to make up for lost time so you have to do more. The recommendation I make to my patients is 45 minutes 5 days a week of INTENTIONAL exercise for general health. This means that just because you walk a lot at work doesn't mean that you are exempt from the exercise requirement. If people are trying to lose weight, I encourage them to do 60 minutes 6 days a week. As an added note, children need 60 minutes a day of moderate to vigorous activity with some sort of muscle building activity included such as sit-ups, pushups, gymnastics, et cetera.

During pregnancy, requirements remain the same. The only slight alteration is that in the 2nd & 3rd trimester, you need to avoid laying on your back because this can cut off blood supply to baby. You also need to avoid doing things like sit ups as this can cause an abdominal hernia due to special hormones that are released that cause your connective tissue to soften in preparation for birth and also so things can stretch with ease (such as your belly). The recommendations remain modified for the first 3 months after delivery as your body goes back to normal.

(CDC: How much physical activity do we need?, n.d.)

(AHA: Recommendations for Physical Activity, 2015)

(WHO: Global Strategy on Diet, Physical Activity and Health, n.d.)

BENEFITS OF EXERCISE BEFORE PREGNANCY

As I have already laid out, exercise is beneficial for your health in general but when it comes to fertility, it can get a little more complicated, too much is bad and too little is bad. If you are exercising a ton, it puts stress on your body and may suppress hormones that help you ovulate. If you are not exercising enough, hormones can also become imbalanced and prevent ovulation. The general guideline when it comes to conception is to follow what the CDC and AHA recommends to the general public (150 minutes) for basic health. Other experts say to do 60 minutes, 6 days a week if you are over-weight but if you are of normal weight and are used to exercising regularly you should limit exercise to 60 minutes per work out session. Underweight women should decrease to about 30 minutes per day and incorporate yoga instead of intense cardio. That being said, recent research shows that women who are in the ideal weight range actually had longer times attempting to conceive if they exercised *vigorously* for more than 5 hours per week with an overall decrease of conception of 42%. The bottom line is that exercise definitely improves your chance of conception by balancing hormones and managing stress but too much can have a negative effect on fertility.

Here is a chart to guide you:

	Vigorous Exercise (running)	Moderate Exercise (jogging/walking)
Ideal Weight (BMI 18.5-24.9)	5 hours or less per week	60 minutes daily
Overweight (BMI >25)	45 minutes 6 days a week	60 minutes 6 days a week
Underweight (BMI <18.5)	30 minutes or less per day	30 minutes or less per day

I want to add here that exercise is important for men as well. Women are not in this alone. Men that don't exercise are at increased risk of low sperm count. And men with a slightly elevated BMI (26-29) are 50% more likely to have problems with fertility. In short, if you are working together to make a baby (as you should) then get to the gym together to increase your odds of conception.

(How Exercise Affects Fertility, 2011)

(Trying to get pregnant? Moderate exercise may help, 2012)

(Fertility 101: Exercise and Fertility, n.d.)

BENEFITS OF EXERCISE DURING PREGNANCY FOR MOM AND BABY

BENEFITS FOR MOM:

Of course, a lot of the benefits are the same such as stress management, improved sleep, improved mood, diabetes prevention, etc. In addition to the regular benefits, it also:

1. Helps your body prepare for labor both mentally and physically—research showed about a two hour decrease in labor time with average labor being just over 6 hours for non-exercisers and just over 4 hours for exercisers. Also, regular exercisers were significantly less likely to request pain meds.
2. Helps improve bowel function to lessen constipation—self-explanatory as exercise stimulates the colon and improves regularity.
3. Helps to decrease back pain commonly associated with pregnancy—women who exercise report less back and pelvic pain than non-exercisers.
4. Helps decrease bloating and swelling that often occurs during pregnancy—by improving blood flow and lymphatic return, you will have less swelling with moderate exercise compared to sedentary mothers.
5. Helps your body bounce back after delivery—research shows women who exercise during pregnancy were able to get back to normal functions quicker than woman who do not exercise.

6. Decreases risk of pregnancy complications—studies showed that women who exercise regularly were less likely to have unplanned C-section (4-fold decrease), forceps delivery (75% less likely) or need an episiotomy (55% less likely).
7. Helps reduce risk of gestational diabetes with an overall decreased incidence of 27%.
8. Decreases morning sickness—although a struggle if you are feeling sick, women who are able to force themselves to exercise have less nausea after a workout compared to those who skip it.
9. Less weight gain and better fitness level later in life—women who exercise during pregnancy had an average weight gain of 7.5 pounds in menopausal years, compared to 22 pounds for non-exercisers. They also found that 20 years after delivery, women who exercised during pregnancy could run two miles 2.5 minutes faster than those who did not.
10. Lowers blood pressure and lessens your chance of pre-eclampsia which is one of the most common causes of premature delivery.

BENEFITS FOR BABY:

It is hard to imagine that your movement would have any benefit on baby but research shows that it most certainly does and the benefits last for a lifetime. Here are some of the top benefits for baby based on rat/mice studies:

1. More optimal birth weight—babies born to mom's who exercised were less likely to be "big babies" and also less likely to be low birth weight babies.
2. Improved insulin sensitivity and therefore decreased risk of diabetes. This was found to continue into adulthood.
3. Decreased risk of neurodegeneration and Alzheimer's. Yes, believe it or not, babies born to mothers who exercised during pregnancy had less brain cell degradation later in life.
4. Improved brain development—Prevention magazine reported a study done by the University of Montreal that showed babies who were tested just a few days (8-12 days old) after birth showed more accelerated brain development by way of sound identification in moms who exercised compared to those that did not.
5. Improved memory and learning abilities: children of mothers who exercise score higher on IQ tests and language tests and have better recall abilities than children of mothers who did not exercise.
6. Less prone to obesity—babies had lower BMI later in life when their moms exercised.
7. Improved heart health—studies showed a slower heart rate in the womb and they found it continued after birth.
8. Improved athleticism later in life—researchers found that young adults performed better in sports if their mothers exercised while they were in the womb.

There are likely more benefits than we can imagine or that science has yet to uncover. The benefits listed here are those that we know about and have been researched. If you are capable of exercise, it is something that you can do, a choice you can make, that will continue to benefit your child well into adulthood. Although we are focused on your two years of sacrifice, I tell all of my patients who are mothers that children learn by example. Making exercise a priority and having your child grow up seeing you exercise on a daily basis will set the stage for them to create a lifetime habit and ritual of regular exercise. As always, if you can't do it for you, do it for your baby.

(13 Benefits of Exericise During Pregnancy , n.d.) (Schlosberg, n.d.) (Domonell, 2013)

(Exercise during pregnancy benefits your baby, 2013)

LIMITATIONS

When it comes to exercise, you have to be smart about what you choose to do. Your body is not the same as it was before you were pregnant. There are biochemical changes, physical changes and positional changes. So, that being said, it probably isn't too surprising that there are some parameters for exercise during pregnancy though such as:

1. Avoid contact sports such as soccer, volleyball, football, et cetera.

2. Avoid heavy lifting as this can harm your body due to the hormones that relax your connective tissue.
3. Avoid twisting motions.
4. Avoid activities that require a lot of balance (especially in 3rd trimester).
5. Avoid interval training (bursts).
6. Avoid activities with the potential to fall such as snowboarding, skiing, horseback riding, et cetera.
7. Avoid abdominal exercises (due to increased risk of abdominal hernia).

Basically, stick to swimming, walking, jogging and doing the elliptical or spin/cycle or similar activities, if you want to err on the side of caution. The general rule of thumb is that if you are already exercising, you can continue to do what you do once you become pregnant as long as it is safe to do so and you don't have any risk factors to prevent you from doing so. Obstetric doctors and midwives will often be overly cautious and tell you not to exercise even with the slightest issue. The top issues that could cause you to slow down are:

1. Bleeding or spotting at any time during pregnancy (discuss with your doctor though as some spotting can be normal early on so the limitations may be lifted in 2nd trimester). However, 2nd & 3rd trimester bleeding is abnormal and will warrant bedrest.

2. Weak cervix—your cervix keeps your baby secure in the womb so if you have been told you have a weak cervix, exercise may not be an option.
3. Signs of premature labor during the current pregnancy.
4. History of premature delivery in previous pregnancies.
5. Active pre-eclampsia.
6. Placenta previa after 26 weeks gestation.
7. Active heart or lung disease.
8. Ruptured membranes.

It is extremely important to discuss any concerns with your doctor. Most of these conditions require bedrest which may be hard for many women. Always ask about swimming as this may be one form of exercise that the body can handle in these circumstances.

(Exercise During Pregnancy, 2015)

(Exercise During Pregancy, n.d.)

(Exerise Benefits, n.d.)

(Exercise During Pregnancy, n.d.)

CHAPTER 9

OTHER LIFESTYLE CONSIDERATIONS

WATER

We live in a society of flavored beverages and the average American is likely extremely dehydrated 100% of the time. Our daily need is half of our body weight in ounces. This means that if you weigh 140 pounds, you need 70 ounces and if you weigh 200 pounds, you need 100 ounces. In addition to the minimum requirement, you need to add an additional ounce for ounce for every caffeinated beverage. If you have 12 ounces of coffee or tea you need an additional 12 ounces of water. Ideally, you would add an additional 16-32 ounces for every hour of cardio/aerobic exercise. These are of course optimal numbers but shooting for half your body weight in ounces should be your minimum. Our bodies are mostly made up of water (60%) and water is required for proper cell function and metabolism. There are many benefits of proper water consumption.

1. Water regulates cellular function—water plays an integral role in pH balance, respiratory function, body temperature and metabolism.
2. Water promotes detoxification—water helps our body detoxify because our kidneys are one of our organs of detoxification so water essentially flushes out the toxins faster.

3. Water keeps skin moist and younger—for obvious reasons, hydrated cells are going to have improved moisture and appear fuller which decreases wrinkles.
4. Water promotes weight loss—when I am recommending weight loss, I encourage people to drink 8-12 ounces of water when they perceive a hunger pain (especially seemingly unwarranted such as one hour after a meal) then wait 10 minutes and see if they are still "hungry". Hunger is often confused with thirst, especially in obesity.
5. Water increases energy—studies show that water improved energy MORE productively than a cup of coffee, especially in that afternoon slump.
6. Water improves muscle function and decreases muscle fatigue—hydrated muscles work better and have less pain so you can use them more efficiently and therefore build muscle more effectively.
7. Water improves mood—The Journal of Nutrition reported a study that showed that cognitive abilities and mood were both muted when the subjects were dehydrated.
8. Water improves brain function—studies show that cognitive function is improved by 30% when people were properly hydrated.
9. Water decreases joint pain—joints are made mostly of water so a dehydrated joint will be painful. Proper hydration therefore decreases pain.

10. Water decreases back pain—low back pain often comes from lack of water and stagnation in that area. Proper water intake can "cure" low back pain. In addition, all of the disks between our vertebrae are composed of primarily water so if a person is not adequately hydrated, they will likely have back pain. Improving water consumption can alleviate this and increase height in some cases!
11. Water decreases risk of osteoporosis—Organicfacts.net reported on a study done by the Linus Pauling institute that showed people who drank proper amounts of water had a decreased risk of developing osteoporosis.
12. Water treats headaches—headaches are often a sign of dehydration.
13. Water treats and prevents constipation—most of water absorption occurs in the colon so if you are dehydrated, water will be pulled out of the colon and therefore leaving you hard stools. Stools without moisture are hard to pass.
14. Water decreases risk of cardiovascular disease and high blood pressure—it dilutes the blood (in a good way) making it thinner and easier to move through the vessels.
15. Water treats and prevents kidney stones—moving fluids through the kidneys helps decrease formation of kidney stones.

(10 health benefits of drinking water) (5 Little Known Benefits of Drinking Water)

(6 Reasons to Drink Water, 2008) (Health Benefits of Drinking Water)

In the realm of fertility, hopefully, the above list makes sense as to why it would help in conception as the body would be functioning better overall. During pregnancy, demands increase due to increased blood volume and the nutrients going to baby. There is also the sac the baby is in that is full of water and requires adequate water intake to maintain. Water also can help prevent pre-eclampsia. During nursing, your body is making upwards of 32 ounces of milk per day which increase your water demands by a full liter so if you are already needing 70 ounces, your now need, 102 ounces at minimum in order to help your body produce milk for your baby.

The next feasible question is whether or not you can just drink tap water out of your sink. The answer is absolutely not! No matter how "clean" they claim municipal water systems are, they are not "clean" by my standards. The reason is quite simple: how do they "clean" the water? With chemicals, of course! Chemicals that the FDA and EPA know exist and test on a regular basis to make sure that the levels don't get too high. I feel like any level of detectable chemicals is too many chemicals, especially for a tiny growing baby. Would you let your kid smoke just one cigarette a day just because it's not as bad as 10? Probably not! In places/municipalities that have less than perfect purification systems, levels of cancer and other health problems are notably higher. A short list includes chlorine, lead (due to pipe corrosion) and some protozoan bacteria that cause gastrointestinal issues. Chlorine is linked to bladder cancer, rectal cancer, breast cancer and asthma. Lead is linked to developmental delays and learning disabilities in children if exposed in the womb and during regular growth and development. There are also pesticides, likely more potent in farming states but present everywhere. There are heavy metals associated with cancer and nervous system issues and benzene which is linked to leukemia. Lastly, there are other chemicals in tap water that cannot be regulated such as pharmaceuticals, cleaning products/byproducts, etc. Basically, your best bet is to purchase a water station (like you would find in an office) and buy a few jugs and fill it at your local grocery store or water vending machine with water that has been treated with reverse osmosis to remove as much of these chemical and byproducts as possible. Then you can fill your glass or stainless-steel containers and have water all day long that you know will not harm you or your baby.

(Wagner) (EPA: Drinking Water Contaminants – Standards and Regulations)

(The Five Most Harmful Chemicals Found in Tap Water, 2009)

(Fluoride and Other Chemicals in Your Drinking Water Could Be Wrecking Your Health, 2013)

WEIGHT

We have discussed exercise and diet but I feel it was worth sharing some facts and statistics about weight that will help motivate you if what you have read so far isn't enough. To start, I will need to define the parameters of weight based on the World Health Organization:

BMI	Category
<16	Extremely underweight
16-17	Moderately Underweight
17-18.5	Mildly Underweight
18.5-25	Normal or ideal weight
25-30	Overweight
30-35	Obese Class I
35-40	Obese Class II
>40	Obese Class III (Morbid Obesity)

(BMI Calculator, n.d.)

Regarding conception, obesity is a risk factor due to its potential to affect ovulation and other factors, some known, some unknown. Since 33% of adults are obese, this is a huge factor in the infertility world. WebMD reported on a study published in the Journal of Human Reproduction that showed the risk of infertility increases even if ovulation is normal in obesity. The study showed that women with BMI over 40 had a 46% less chance of conception and women with a BMI that lands between 35 and 40 had 26% less chance of conception in the reported study.

There are two categories of fertility problems in women who are obese:

1. Ovulating
2. Non-Ovulating

The cause of infertility in obese women who have normal ovulation is unclear but it is speculated that it is related to elevated leptin levels (leptin regulates hunger & satiety) and low adiponectin levels (adiponectin regulates fat and blood sugar levels). Although the cause is unknown, the good news is that decreasing weight by 5-10% (about a 30-pound loss in a 300-pound woman) significantly increases the chances of conception. With the two-year sacrifice in mind, this can be achieved in a relatively short period of time although your window of sacrifice may be longer as this type of weight loss will take some time (probably about 4 months).

As for non-ovulating women, infertility is usually related to a condition called PCOS or Polycystic Ovary Syndrome. These women often have a myriad of issues including irregular menstrual cycles, elevated LH, elevated testosterone, elevated DHEA, elevated cholesterol and insulin resistance and resulting anovulation. (It is important to note that not all women with PCOS are obese and also not all obese women have PCOS and lastly, not all women with PCOS have all of the issues listed). Conception can be rather challenging for these women as they do not ovulate. It is my experience that the best way to manage PCOS is through diet and exercise but it often requires use of pharmaceuticals such as Metformin or Spironolactone to help manage insulin and androgen levels to make ovulation possible.

In addition to having trouble conceiving, obesity increases the rate of miscarriage and it is speculated that it is related to poorer quality of eggs, defective egg implantation due to insulin resistance and altered hormone levels that help maintain pregnancy once established. In referencing earlier sections on food additives and chemicals, there may be more to it that we realize. It may not just be obesity that is causing these but more so the foods that are consumed to sustain a higher BMI that are full of toxins, endocrine disruptors and other disease-causing chemicals.

As I have mentioned throughout this book, this issue is not all on the female. Obesity affects male fertility as well. Carolina Conceptions reports on a study that showed men in the overweight category (BMI 26-28) had a 50% decline in fertility with an even higher incidence if men are in the obese category. Excess fat causes a rise in estrogen which lowers sperm counts. It also increases the temperature of the scrotum which results in lower count and quality of sperm. WebMD reported a more specific Danish study that showed BMI over 25 caused a decrease in sperm count by 24% and decrease in sperm concentration by 22% and a measurable decrease in testosterone levels. So, ladies, remember that baby making is a team effort and takes multiple ingredients. You don't want to bake bread with good eggs but rotten flour or vice versa because either way, it's not going to be as good as it could be and the goal here is to strive to do the best we can in the mastering the recipe for the perfect baby.

One additional note, on the day that I was putting my finishing touches on this book, I happened to have The Today Show on for the December 3, 2015 episode and they were reporting on research that showed as little as a 6-pound weight gain between your first pregnancy and your second pregnancy can increase your chances of a stillborn baby by 50%. The probability is low in general but absolutely higher for women with obesity and they found a definite correlation to not losing the baby weight from the first pregnancy and the health of the second pregnancy. The report emphasized the importance of maintaining a healthy weight for conception and pregnancy.

(Boyles, 2007) (Dr Ananya Mandal, n.d.)
(Fertility 101: Exercise and Fertility, n.d.)

(Obesity Takes a Toll on Sperm and Fertility, 2004)

SLEEP

Most people love to sleep but the majority of American's do not get enough. I recommend a minimum of 7 hours per night for men and 8 hours per night for women. Of course, individual needs may vary but those are the basic recommendation that I make to my patients. The reasoning for these hours is that the purpose of sleep is for DNA repair and replication and this process takes about 6 hours. So, if you are falling short of your requirement, it is like stopping the assembly line early and compromising cellular restoration. Chronic sleep deprivation can, in my opinion, ultimately lead to cancer as a result of impaired DNA repair leaving it vulnerable to mutation. In relation to fertility, lack of sleep can affect ALL the hormones related to ovulation such as estrogen, FSH, LH and progesterone, as well as leptin levels which also affect ovulation along with hunger and satiety. The Huffington Post reported a study that showed women undergoing IVF, who got 7-8 hours had the highest rate of successful pregnancy at 53% compared to 46% in those who got 4-6 hours. Interesting to note though is that they also studied women who got 9-11 hours of sleep and their pregnancy rate was 43%! So, as with most things, you CAN get too much of a good thing and everything should be executed or accomplished in moderation!

Our normal sleep-wake cycle is controlled by a circadian rhythm. Normal functioning of that circadian rhythm affects our hormones. Shift workers have an altered circadian rhythm and there is documented research that shift workers have a higher incidence of miscarriage. If you are trying to get pregnant and are currently working a shift work schedule (particularly 3rd shift), you should try to request a change, even if for a short period of time. This also applies to your spouse. Sleep deprivation and altered circadian rhythm can cause a lower sperm count. Sleep deprivation has also been linked to erectile dysfunction, lowered immune system, depression, low libido and many other issues (including obesity, high blood pressure, insulin resistance and altered cortisol (stress hormone) levels).

(Put the Sleep and Infertility Link to Rest, n.d.)

(Sleep, Fertility Linked: 7-8 Hours Best For IVF Patients, Study Says, 2013)

(Effects of Sleep Deprivation on Fertility, n.d.)

Sleep is critical to your health, whether you are trying to get pregnant, trying to grow a baby or trying to deal with the demands of life. In addition to my Basic Food Tips, all my new patients also get a Sleep Well Tips handout. It is a guide on how to get optimal sleep.

Sleep Hygiene

1. Establish Routine: work on going to bed at the same time every day but more importantly, getting up at the same time every day.
2. Limit caffeine: caffeine should be limited to morning time only, if at all and none after 2pm (Yes! Including green tea!)

3. Television: remove the TV from the bedroom. The bedroom should be reserved for sleeping and intimate moments only.
4. Prepare to sleep: do not watch television, read a suspense novel, surf the internet and try not to argue with your spouse/partner for 30-60 minutes before bed. This will decrease stimulating or disturbing thoughts or images as you try to go to sleep. Before bed, dim the house lights and try to do something relatively "mindless" like dishes, folding laundry or quality time with your spouse, kids or pets.
5. Food: try not to eat two hours before bed as digestion takes away from the restorative processes that need to take place while you sleep. If you must eat chose primarily protein sources such as a slice of turkey or nuts.
6. Quiet: don't listen to music or the radio while sleeping. Sound keeps your brain active and therefore, out of deep sleep and rest. If you need music to fall asleep, make sure you use a "sleep function" so it will turn off after 15-30 minutes. If you live in a situation where noise is inevitable (your partner snores, there are trains every half-hour, et cetera), try earplugs. Other things that can help are double paned windows, heavy drapes, or rugs on hardwood. Consider a quite oscillating fan for a little "white noise" but keep in mind that if it is too loud, it will actually keep you out of the deep restorative sleep.

7. Cool: Make sure the room is cool. If you can, open the window. It's ok to pile on the blankets but the room temperature should be cool. If you have a time controlled thermostat, have it drop down to 66 degrees about an hour before bed.
8. Electric blankets: NO! We are energetic beings and sleeping under an electric current is not healthy for our sleep cycle, even if it is off as the current is still pulsing through the wires if it is plugged in! Get a down comforter and put extra blankets on top if you get cold easily. If you feel like you can't live without your electric blanket, I suggest using it to heat up your bed then turn it off and unplug it from the foot of the bed or from the wall to stop the current from circulating over you all night.
9. Darkness: Make sure the room is dark...really dark. Turn cell phones upside down if they charge in your bedroom, put a small towel over your digital clock or get a new one altogether that doesn't illuminate the room. No nightlights, candles, etc.
10. Air Quality: as stated before, open the window if possible. Do not have any chemical air fresheners in your bedroom, as they are toxic in general but definitely not to be breathed in an enclosed room for 8 hours.
11. Animals: ideally animals shouldn't be in the room with you at all but that is not always feasible so try to keep them off the bed to reduce allergies and avoid "space occupying nuisances".
12. Sheets: clean sheets weekly to reduce dust and allergens.

13. Environment: as stated above, the environment is important to your sleep hygiene. Keep your room as clean as possible, free of dust and allergens. Keep your bedroom door closed during the day with your window slightly opened. Turn your phone on to "airplane mode" to decrease EMF toxicity and remove all other electronics from the bedroom.
14. Exercise: If possible, try not to partake in vigorous exercise within 2-4 hours of bedtime as it increases endorphins, which may keep you in a state of arousal. Some people find exercise to be helpful for sleep so do what works for you.
15. Try a hot bath or shower to relax the body.
16. Try relaxation exercises to train your body to relax and your mind to let go when you get in bed. For example, lay perfectly still and put your body parts to sleep one by one from the bottom, up (i.e. "my foot is completely relaxed...my ankle is completely relaxed...and so on). Make yourself start over if you get fidgety or stray in your thoughts. Or try deep breathing—ten second inhale, ten second exhale.
17. If you still cannot sleep, you should consider getting a referral for a sleep study, there may be organic reasons for your restlessness.

ALCOHOL

I could not write a book on conception and pregnancy and not discuss alcohol. There is information everywhere, even posted in bars and on some beverages that alcohol can harm your baby. Remember we are talking about the two-year sacrifice here so the best option is to avoid it altogether as there is no known safe amount to drink during pregnancy. The possible effects are irreversible and range from physical deformities to learning disabilities. Children with Fetal Alcohol Syndrome are mentally, emotionally and physically deformed and have a lifelong struggle as a result, including a large percentage of them ending up in prison due to problems with judgement and inability to differentiate between right and wrong and also lacking discernment in social cues.

From the moment of conception, your baby starts developing and within just over two weeks, the heart is forming and by week 3, the brain starts to develop. So, if you are reading this in preparation of pregnancy, it would be ideal to stop drinking, at least on the second half of your cycles (from ovulation to the start of the next period). If you are already pregnant, hopefully you have stopped drinking but if you haven't, now is the time. Alcohol is known to contribute to miscarriage and premature birth and some studies have shown a 70% increased risk of having a still born baby if you drink 5 drinks per week while pregnant.

Many people argue that people in Europe continue to drink throughout pregnancy and their babies are fine but the World Health Organization reported on a study that showed there are measurable behavioral, emotional, hyperactivity and attention differences in children age 3-5 whose mothers drank 1-4 drinks per week during pregnancy. That same research found there were no significant differences past age 5 in non-drinkers vs light drinkers. TIME magazine reported on a study that was published in the International Journal of Obstetrics and Gynecology that studied over 10,000 7-year old children in the UK and found no difference in behavioral or cognitive ability when comparing children from mothers who drank light amounts of alcohol versus no alcohol. Although a study published a few years prior (2007) in the journal called Pediatrics, they reported an opposite finding in a similar study with only one drink per week affecting behavior in girls age 4-8 years of age. In recent years, several European countries have started to follow in the footsteps of the United States due to increases in Fetal Alcohol Syndrome. The UK alone reports about 6,000 incidences per year, while the US reports about 40,000 cases per year.

As far as pre-conception goes, alcohol can also affect your chances of getting pregnant. Alcohol depletes vitamins and minerals so it can affect you and your partner adversely if you are trying to conceive. It also bogs down the liver which can interfere with hormone metabolism and cause a build-up of estrogen which can cause infertility (see chart from the Balancing Hormones section) for both women and men. For men, alcohol depletes vitamin C which is required to keep sperm from clumping together. Vitamin C also protects the DNA inside of the sperm so essentially, alcohol decreases the quality of genetic material that is contributed by dad. So, if you are in the window of trying to conceive, abstaining from alcohol as a couple, would be advised if you want the best possible odds as well as the best possible genetic material.

The bottom line is that heavy drinking during pregnancy absolutely does cause Fetal Alcohol Syndrome and light drinking may or may not cause behavioral or cognitive impairment. In an effort to grow the "perfect baby", it is best to hold out for this short period of time when there are too many unknowns and you never want to look back and wonder if something you did caused an issue with your baby's development. Alcohol also affects your fertility and your partner's fertility as well as the quality of sperm and egg that come together. Your spouse/partner is off the hook once you are pregnant but ask him to help you through this journey by limiting his consumption or abstaining altogether during this precious time.

(Alcohol and Pregnancy: Is 'A Little Bit' Safe?, n.d.)

(Alcohol Use in Pregnancy, n.d.) (Alcohol Use During Pregnancy, n.d.)

(Pregnancy and Alcohol, 2015)

(Is low does alcohol exposure during pregnancy harmful, 2010)

(Graff, 2009) (Yang, 2013) (Infertility and Alcohol, n.d.) (Alcohol & Fertility, n.d.)

SMOKING

This is another area that can't be ignored. It is surprising to say that although there is a plethora of information out there and warnings come on almost all packages of cigarettes that they cause low birth weight, premature birth and birth defects (cleft palate in particular), there are still an astounding number of women who smoke during pregnancy, almost 1 in 4. Obviously, people want to turn a blind eye to reality but smoking still kills thousands of people per year. Part of the detrimental effects from cigarettes are due to the 599 chemicals (give or take depending on the brand) that are ADDED to tobacco to make them burn quicker, smell better, be more addictive, control negative effects from smoking, etc. Several of these chemicals can be found in the toxic food additives list already discussed previously. In addition to these added toxic chemicals, when they are lit or burned, additional chemical reactions take place producing byproduct chemicals with totals varying from 4000 to 7000 depending on your source.

As far as conception is concerned, smoking does interfere with your fertility, mostly due to the plethora of chemicals that go into your body with each cigarette. Those chemicals damage your ovaries, damage your eggs, and they even damage your genetic material! It is also one of the top causes of miscarriage which is also a fertility issue. As per usual, it is not all on the woman to quit—smoking causes low sperm count, hormone disruption in men and decreased erectile function. In addition, second hand smoke may be as harmful to you as smoking yourself as far as fertility is concerned. The chemicals added to cigarettes are potent enough to linger in the air and get into your body even if they are not directly inhaled. A lot of people decide they will quit as soon as they find out they are pregnant but to optimize your genetic material and your chance of creating a "perfect baby", it is best to quit when you know you are going to start trying to make a baby.

During pregnancy, as I have already stated, babies born to smoking mothers have risk of low birth weight, premature delivery and physical birth defects such as cleft palate as well as cerebral palsy and mental retardation. There is evidence that babies born to mothers who smoke during pregnancy have several other issues that affect long term health and development. Here is a list:

1. Lower IQ and learning disabilities. One study reported that there is a 25% increase in having dyslexia when mother's smoke during pregnancy.
2. Obesity and diabetes affects more adults later in life if their mothers smoked while they were in the womb. Specifically, there was a higher incidence of Type 2 diabetes with onset prior to age 33 which is considered early onset Type 2 diabetes.
3. Elevated blood pressure was found in children around 5-6 years of age whose mothers smoked compared to children at the same age. This

propensity towards hypertension carried into adulthood as well.

4. Behavioral problems such as impulsivity and a higher likelihood to engage in criminal behaviors including drug use. Retroactive studies that determined this link took into account socioeconomic status thus confirming the link to in utero exposure to cigarettes and the likelihood of behavioral issues.
5. Respiratory problems; these children have an increased risk of asthma later in life.
6. Sudden Infant Death syndrome risk is increased by 2-3-fold.
7. Congenital Heart Defect incidence was increased in women who smoked the first trimester by as much as 20 to 70%.

In summary, smoking during pregnancy is clearly not a good idea. If you are reading this and still smoking, it is never too late to stop. I would say this about the entire book really. Knowledge is power and when, in your journey, you obtain that knowledge is not always in your control. Once you have the knowledge however, it is your responsibility to protect your baby, even against your strongest addictions.

Many women want to know if they can smoke after the baby is born but before you light up again, you should know that second hand smoke definitively harms your child and can increase risk of asthma and lung cancer as well as leukemia due to benzene (one of the chemicals in second hand smoke). There is research that confirms children exposed to ongoing second-hand smoke have higher incidences of infections, especially respiratory infections such bronchitis and pneumonia. Then you could just smoke outside, right? Well, in addition to second hand smoke causing disease, infection and cancer in your baby, there is now something called "third hand smoke". The idea of this concept is often shocking to many people but might make sense to others. Third hand smoke is the toxic residue from smoking that remains on hair, skin and clothing. There is evidence that even third hand smoke can be almost as harmful as second-hand smoke. Current research links third hand smoke to respiratory illness, ear infections and even decline in cognitive abilities and IQ.

In summary, there is never a safe time to smoke when it comes to you or your baby. Even after the two-year window of sacrifice, you can see that smoking is something that can continue to affect your baby well beyond this window I have laid out. To optimize your child's development and overall health, smoking should be considered a non-negotiable for both mom and dad.

(Tobacco Use and Pregnancy, n.d.) (Smoking & Infertility, n.d.)

(Michael Rabinoff, 2007, Nov) (Long-Term Effects of Tobacco on a Fetus, 2015)

(Smoking During Pregnancy, 2015) (Woolston, n.d.)

(Second Hand Smoke, 2015) (Third Hand Smoke a Danger to Babies, Toddlers, 2010)

(Markel, 2009) (Ballantyne, 2009) (Smoking during pregnancy, 2014)

LEGAL AND ILLEGAL DRUGS, NON-PRESCRIPTION

I am not going to spend much time on this subject, in fact, I nearly forgot to include it. My reasoning is that if you purchased this book and are currently reading this book, I am guessing that you are probably not doing drugs. This is a no brainer subject for most people who are actually making an effort to get pregnant so the percentage of readers who are likely to skip this section is pretty high but the book would not be complete without discussing drugs & pregnancy as some are now legal. Not to mention the fact that perhaps someone bought the book FOR you in hopes that you will make better choices for you and your baby. So, if that is the case, I will give a quick run-down of detrimental effects of drugs before, during and after pregnancy for you or for anyone who is interested in the subject.

Cannabis/Marijuana

Preconception/Fertility Problems: Increase risk of miscarriage, decreased LH production/release thus leading to ovulation problems in women and also there is slowing of movement of the egg through the fallopian tube thus decreasing chance of implantation. In men, they have decreased sperm counts.

Effects during pregnancy: Still born birth.

Short-term effects on baby: Low birth weight babies and newborns are unsettled and startle more easily. There is also and increase risk of SIDS. Some withdrawal symptoms such as excessive crying and tremors

Long Term effects on baby: Learning disabilities, impaired memory & behavioral issues such as impulsivity and ADD

Methamphetamines/Amphetamines/Ecstacy

Preconception/Fertility Problems: Increase risk of miscarriage

Effects during pregnancy: Placetal insufficiency, placental abruption, premature birth

Short-term effects on baby: Low birth weight and withdrawal symptoms at birth, increase risk of SIDS

Long Term effects on baby: Impaired development, behavioral issues and learning disabilities. Impaired motor skills and impaired coordination, life-long impairment in vision, hearing and breathing.

Cocaine/Crack

Preconception/Fertility Problems:

In men, it causes low sperm count and poor sperm quality.

In women, it can disrupt the menstrual cycle inhibiting ovulation. It also increases prolactin which causes hormone imbalances with the other primary female hormones.

It also can cause scarring and permanent damage to the fallopian tubes.

If pregnancy occurs, there is an increased risk of miscarriage.

Effects during pregnancy: Placental abruption, membrane rupture, premature delivery or fetal death. Increase risk correlation to cleft palate.

Birth defects in multiple organs, systems and structures including skull, face, eyes, arms, legs, heart, intestines, reproductive organs including genitals and urinary system.

Short-term effects on baby: Low birth weight, risk of death in first month of life and they have sensory problems such as irritability, tremors, poor sleep, visual disturbances and stimulation issues.

Long Term effects on baby: Learning and behavioral issues

Opiates: Heroine/Morphine/Tramadol

Preconception/Fertility Problems:

Affects menstrual cycle, usually causing it to stop altogether.

If pregnancy occurs, increased risk of miscarriage

Effects during pregnancy: Membrane rupture and premature birth, stillborn, stunted brain development

Short-term effects on baby: Low Birth Weight, respiratory challenges (difficulty breathing) and withdrawal symptoms

Long Term effects on baby: Behavioral problems, developmental delays, possible growth retardation and lower IQ

Hallucinogens (LSD, PCP, Ecstasy, Mushrooms, etc)

Preconception/Fertility Problems: None specific to this category

Effects during pregnancy: PCP is known to cause skeletal dysplasia, facial abnormalities, skull deformities, and central nervous system deficiencies, abnormalities in other organ systems such as heart, lungs, urinary system and musculoskeletal systems as well as cleft palate. Other drugs in this category have not shown detrimental effects on the fetus. LSD may cause defects of arms and legs, heart defects, and visual defects.

Short-term effects on baby: Babies from mother's who used PCP usually show withdrawal symptoms similar to opioid use such as tremors, irritability, jitters, digestive disturbances, etc.

Long Term effects on baby: Ecstasy has demonstrated impaired motor skills and impaired coordination

(Illegal Drugs in Pregnancy, 2013)

(Illegal drugs and their affect on your fertility, 2013) (Pardes, 2014)

(Drug Babies and the Effects of Drug Abuse During Pregnancy, n.d.)

(Christopher Dvorak, Carrie L. McMahon, & Eugene Pergament, 2000)

CAFFEINE

Considering how most people live life these days, mentioning a decrease or elimination of caffeine is nearly sacrilegious. So, as with everything, I am here to present the facts and you ultimately get to choose. You are reading this book because you are interested in creating a "perfect baby" so I suppose if you love your coffee too much, you may decide to lower your bar of perfection. That being said, it is not just coffee that has us wrapped around its little finger. There are many sources of caffeine other than coffee. Coffee just happens to be one of the more natural sources. If you are a soda drinker, I want to reference you back to the section on food additives so you can combine that knowledge with what you are about to read. I will start by giving you a breakdown of caffeine content so that the reports make sense. There were many sources demonstrating various levels of caffeine so I opted to use Starbucks and Mayo Clinic's breakdown for the sake of credibility. I will leave out some as to spare extra details but I will say that "decaffeinated" beverages that are caffeinated by nature, do have some amounts of caffeine, usually under 5mg. Regarding coffee beans and tea leaves, many people feel that the decaffeination process is much more harmful than just drinking the natural caffeine due to the many chemicals required to get the caffeine out.

Here is what Starbucks and Mayo Clinic report for caffeine content:

SOURCE	MEASURE	CAFFEINE CONTENT
Brewed coffee	8 ounces	95-200mg
Brewed, Keurig pod	8 ounces	75-150mg
Starbucks Drip	16 ounces	300-360mg
Frappuccino	16 ounces	90-110mg
Espresso	1 shot	47-75mg
Instant coffee	8 ounces	27-173mg
Black Tea	8 ounces	14-74mg
Green Tea	8 ounces	24-45mg
Bottle Iced tea	8 ounces	5-40mg
Most Soda	12 ounces	23-55mg
Energy Drinks	8 ounces	70-100mg

(Nutrition and Healthy Eating: Caffeine content for coffee, tea, soda and more, 2014)

(Caffeine Content in Starbucks Beverages, n.d.)

Caffeine, Pre-conception and Fertility:

Caffeine absolutely does affect your ability to conceive. It actually hampers the ability of the fallopian tube to move the egg down the line towards the uterus thus decreasing possibility of implantation in time. Fertility Authority reported on a study from the 80's done by Yale that showed a 55% increased risk of infertility in women who drank just one cup of coffee per day. The risk continued to increase with increased consumption with 1-3 cups yielding a 100% increased risk and over 3 cups showing a 176% increased risk. The same source reported a study done by Kaiser that showed a two fold increase in miscarriages in women who drank about 1.5 cups of coffee per day or 200mg of caffeine (from any source). Optimizing Fertility published an article that was originally published in 2009 in Resolve for the Journey and Beyond, that reported even small amounts of caffeine decreased the incidence of live birth and that animal studies have shown that caffeine interferes with the formation of the egg (oocyte).

(The Effects of Caffeine on Fertility, n.d.)

(Samuel A. Pauli, 2009)

Caffeine Effects on Your Baby

If you were not one of the women who was unfortunately affected by caffeine when you were trying to conceive and you are now pregnant, the next bit of information is for you. Hands down, caffeine can cause low birth weight. Livestrong reported on studies that showed an association between caffeine and neural tube defects, cleft palate and even undescended testes in boys. Animal studies show a correlation between caffeine consumption and physical birth defects, heart defects, preterm labor and delivery and babies born with low birth weight. At birth, babies born to mothers who were drinking caffeine were harder to console, had increased heart rate and a greater startle response. In addition, the Journal of Clinical Nutrition reports decrease in skeletal growth of fetuses born to mothers who consume caffeine.

There may also be cognitive and behavioral consequences but this is somewhat unknown and hard to study due to many other potential factors. A study published in Behavioral Brain Research in 2009, found a correlation to prenatal exposure to caffeine and cognitive changes that lasted into adulthood, especially related to memory. Related behavioral changes were discounted in the Academy of Pediatrics; however, an earlier study in 1988 done on rats showed significant consequences to brain development and behavior including hyperactivity, learning disabilities and increased food consumption later in life. Additionally, a study done in 1990 showed that low dose caffeine caused decreased emotions and increased activity but high dose caffeine caused increased emotions and decreased activity. Most of the rat studies showed males being more susceptible to these changes in development and behavior. Finally, the best article I found in my research was essentially a meta-analysis of most of the studies that showed detrimental effects of caffeine (including Sudden Infant Death Syndrome!). In his summary, Jean-Paul Marat concludes that due to the research available that demonstrates measurable harm to rat babies and the possibility that early exposure to caffeine may be linked to SIDS and possibly disease later in life, caffeine should be avoided during pregnancy. I definitely agree with his conclusion and I find it interesting that all the negative research reported occurred in the 80's and 90's but since what I would call, the "Coffeehouse Revolution" occurred in the US in the mid to late 1990's, suddenly there is a blind eye to one of our most commonly used and socially acceptable drugs of choice. In addition, it is interesting to note that according to the CDC, from the years of 1997 to 2006, the diagnosis of ADHD increased by 3% per year but since 2006, it increases by 5% per year and ironically (or not so ironically), boys are more likely to be diagnosed than girls. This finding aligns with the findings that susceptibility was more prominent in males as reported in rat studies. I personally believe that there is a hands down correlation to maternal caffeine intake and behavior later in life. As I opened this section with, this information leaves you with a decision to make; to weigh out your desires over your baby's health and future struggles, founded or unfounded but by correlation and chance.

(Stephanie Draus, 2013)

(Caffeine during pregnancy, 2015) (Caffeine during pregnancy, 2005)

(Bakker R, 2010 June) (Deborah E. Soellner, 2009)

(Eva M. Loomans, August 2012) (Friedera, 1988, Vol 41, Issue 1-2)

(Hughes & Beveridge, 1990) (ADHD: New Data: Medication and Behavior, 2015)

CHAPTER 10

SUPPLEMENTS

In all my new patient folders, I include a handout on basic supplementation which is a list of vitamins and nutrients I feel every person needs to move towards optimal health. Vitamins and minerals are required for the regulation of the body's basic metabolic functions. They are found naturally in many of the foods that we eat and are also added to many processed foods in the name of "fortification". There are two types of vitamins: water soluble and fat soluble, which means some are processed through you and excreted in urine and some require fat to be absorbed and they are then stored in fat. There are only four fat soluble vitamins (A, D, E, K) and the rest are water soluble. The fat-soluble vitamins can become toxic but it takes very high doses for prolonged periods of time before signs of toxicity begin to show up.

My recommendation is usually high dose supplementation, especially of the water-soluble vitamins. Fat soluble vitamins can be used in high doses but need to be monitored by a physician (by checking blood levels with a laboratory) in most cases. My reasoning for high dose supplementation is that even if you have what you would consider an optimal diet, our soils are depleted and it is challenging to get what we need from a whole foods diet. Many argue that foods are fortified so you can get your vitamins from those sources but that implies you are eating processed foods which I don't suggest in general but especially not to sustain health to avoid swallowing a few pills. In addition to those reasons, no two humans are the same and even the same human will have different needs on a day to day basis. Our needs change based on how much sleep we get, how much exercise we perform, how much stress we are under, how much and which foods we eat, how many toxins we take in, how much caffeine or alcohol we drink and many other factors. If you give high dose supplements, the body can use what it needs at that particular time and get rid of the rest. Getting the minimum is not enough for optimal health. I call the RDA/DV the "BMTS" which is the Bare Minimum To Survive and avoid disease because that is exactly what it is. These levels laid out by the government are the minimum requirements to prevent disease. For example, we need 60mg of Vitamin C to prevent scurvy, we need 800IU of Vitamin D to prevent rickets and so on. I explain to my patients that I want you to do more than just SURVIVE! I want you to THRIVE! There are many people that are ok with just surviving and getting by but most of the people that come to see me want more from their healthcare and they strive for improved health, not just sustainability. I hope that you are one of those people too.

All of the general information above is in relation to a regular human being who is looking to improve health. If you are reading this, you are looking to make a baby or optimize your baby's health in the womb and after delivery into their life. I will first discuss each primary nutrient and its benefit for your knowledge base. Then, I generally modify my list of essentials as the pregnancy progresses based on where the baby's development is so I will break it down into conception, trimesters and breast feeding. I also want to take a moment to discuss QUALITY of supplements. Finding the cheapest supplement will not serve you well. It may not have what it says it has, the specified nutrient may not be present in the quantity specified or it may not be in an absorbable form. I encourage use of capsules over tablets as they are easier to absorb. Purchase your supplements from a credible source and look for "Pharmaceutical Grade" whenever possible. Pharmaceutical Grade means that they have been assayed to confirm that they have what the manufacturer says they have in them, usually by an outside source. Some good brands are Vital Nutrients, Pure Encapsulations, Nordic Naturals, Vitanica, Thorne, Integrative Therapeutics to name a few.

BASIC SUPPLEMENTATION

VITAMIN/ NUTRIENT	**BENEFICIAL EFFECTS**
PRENATAL MULTIVITAMIN For Men: MULTIVITAMIN	This should be a comprehensive multivitamin that covers your basis and usually has a modest dose of vitamins (not too high, not too low) with extra folate and usually a little extra iron as well. It has lower doses of Vitamin A (which causes birth defects) and usually in the form of beta carotene to increase safety. A good one will have a balance

	of copper and zinc, a modest dose of iodine and selenium to help your thyroid. This is tough to hear, but it is better to get one that you have to take several of per day as they are less likely to make you feel nauseated and more likely to be absorbed. Favorite Brand: Vital Nutrients
OMEGA 3 FATTY ACID	I could write a whole book on the benefits of omega 3 fatty acids. In general, Omega 3 helps prevent heart disease and cancer, it helps manage rheumatoid arthritis, decreases inflammation, helps treat depression, improves lung function in asthmatics, decreases symptoms of ADHD and helps prevent Alzheimer's and dementia. Specific to the topics in this book, I will say for preconception, it decreases inflammation first and foremost which will help prepare the body for conception. For the baby, it improved brain development, increases IQ, improves communication and social development, and improves sensory development and motor development. Favorite Brands: Nordic Naturals and Xymogen

	(What to know about Omega 3's and Fish, n.d.) (Omega 3 Fatty Acids Fact Sheet, n.d.) (Omega-3 Intake During Last Months Of Pregnancy Boosts An Infant's Cognitive And Motor Development, 2008)
B COMPLEX	B Vitamins are found in nearly every biochemical reaction in your cells, especially in relation to creating cellular energy. They each have a specific function. In general, they are required for energy, metabolism, brain function, vision, tissue repair, digestion, cellular growth, nervous system regulation, protein building, red blood cell maintenance and DNA repair and regeneration. So, as you can see, this is a non-negotiable requirement! Our B vitamin needs definitely fall into that category of variable needs especially in regard to stress levels. Favorite Brands: Vital Nutrients and Pure Encapsulations
VITAMIN C	This is my favorite anti-oxidant because it is so well-rounded. There are lots of antioxidant choices out there but this one gets the gold medal for multiple benefits. In addition to being an antioxidant (which means in decreases free-radicals that cause cancer), it helps

	with tissue repair, cartilage building, oral/dental health, vascular integrity, helps with iron absorption and helps with healing after surgery, trauma or burns. I like to mix it up with capsules from Vital Nutrients and chewable tablets from Natural Factors. Favorite Brands: Vital Nutrients and Natural Factors (Vitamin C, n.d.)
VITAMIN D	Vitamin D is essential for bone growth and protection as it aids in calcium absorption. It also improves the immune system, boosts mood and helps treat muscle weakness. I have seen chronic, life-long depression completely resolve with adequate vitamin D supplementation. Other common uses include prevention and treatment of cancer & autoimmune disease, PMS, asthma, psoriasis and a plethora of other conditions. Our main source is from the sun but I have met residents of Maui, Hawaii with vitamin D deficiency. You have to go outside every single day right around noon, without sunscreen and have exposed skin in order to get your body's minimal requirement. In a

	conference I recently attended, they mentioned that blood levels below 60 do not give benefits beyond bone health. I have always worked towards and optimal blood level of 60-80ng/mL Favorite Brands: Vital Nutrients and Pure Encapsulations (Professional Monographs, n.d.)
CALCIUM/ MAGNESIUM	Calcium has gotten some bad press recently but it is still one of my loves and my thought is that a couple of negative studies should not discount years of positive research. Also, it is my theory that the problem is not from calcium supplements, it is from excess intake of dairy and fortified/processed foods. It is easy to get too much if you are having 3-5 (or more!) servings of dairy PLUS adding in a supplement. Calcium is not only for your bones. I use it for colon cancer prevention, muscle cramping & electrolyte balance. Other practitioners use it for PMS, pre-eclampsia, and a host of other conditions. I never give calcium alone, it is always in a complex with magnesium and other nutrients. Calcium citrate is the most absorbable form. Magnesium is one of most depleted

	nutrients in our body yet it is required for healthy bones and teeth, optimal nervous system function, cardiovascular function, muscle transmission and relaxation and energy metabolism. I use it for anxiety, high blood pressure, insomnia, kidney stones, migraines, restless leg, arrhythmia, fibromyalgia, constipation and many other conditions. **I like to take these two in combination to decrease the number of pills. If I am treating a specific condition, I will add a specific form of magnesium in addition to a calcium complex. Favorite Brands: Vital Nutrients (OsteoNutrients II) and Twin Labs TriBoron Plus (not a pharmaceutical grade but a fantastic formula) (Professional Monographs, n.d.)
"FOLIC ACID" aka FOLATE OR METHYLFOLATE	I will discuss this more in detail in Mixing the Batter below but for now we will discuss the importance of folate in general health and of course before and during pregnancy. Folate is used for anemia, oral/dental issues such as gum disease and canker sores, memory problems and dementia prevention, cervical dysplasia, cervical

	cancer, restless leg, cardiovascular disease and multiple other acute and chronic diseases. For pregnancy, it is used to prevent neural tube defects and is ideally taken and higher doses for a full year before conception. Neural tube defect is incomplete closure of the spinal cord or skull during early development of the baby (in the first few weeks of pregnancy). This defect can be somewhat benign (barely noticeable) or tragically fatal (anencephaly). Folate also prevents defects such as cleft palate and some congenital heart defects. It is also known to prevent pre-eclampsia which occurs later in pregnancy so it is advised to take this before and throughout pregnancy. Favorite Brands: Xymogen, Biogenesis (Professional Monographs, n.d.) (folic acid: why you need it before and during pregnancy, n.d.)
PROBIOTICS	I have really become passionate about probiotics in the last couple of years and only recently added it to my Basic Supplementation handout. I have learned more and more about how gut health and balanced gut flora can affect

	almost every aspect of your health from your teeth and gums to your mood and brain function. It is known to decrease tooth decay, lower LDL cholesterol (the bad one), improve digestion (BOTH diarrhea AND constipation) and decreases gas, bloating and abdominal discomfort, improves eczema, improve vaginal health, improve respiratory health & immunity (it can lower your chance of getting sick!), and decreases infant crying (what!?). Another study reported that children born to women who took probiotics during pregnancy had a 30% less chance of having eczema and ultimately less chance of allergies later. It also boosts immunity, helps with acne, and helps with weight loss. People think you can get what you need from yogurt but that is an extremely low dose and I recommend capsules and at least 10 billion per capsule if not more. Favorite Brands: Orthomolecular, Klaire Labs, Xymogen and Pure Encapsulations (Maier, 2013) (Melnick, 2012)

OTHER NUTRIENTS

VITAMIN/NUTRIENT	BENEFICIAL EFFECTS
VITEX / CHASTE TREE	Stimulates the release of LH and modulates progesterone levels. Favorite Brand: Pure Encapsulations—Vitex 750
RHODIOLA	Improves adrenal function and thyroid function and helps with egg maturation. Favorite Brands: Vital Nutrients and Pure Encapsulations
VITAMIN E Mixed Tocopherols	An antioxidant that helps treat cardiovascular disease, angina, hypertension, BPH, cancer, diabetes and many more. It also helps improve sperm quality thus improving fertility in men. And in women it helps modulate hormones and improves symptoms of PMS, dysmenorrhea, miscarriages and infertility with an uncertain mechanism. It can also help prevent and treat pre-eclampsia. Favorite Brands: Vital Nutrients and Pure Encapsulations
SELENIUM	An antioxidant which helps improve sperm count and quality and maximizes testosterone. In women, it can help regulate the

	thyroid and in turn improve fertility. (Improved thyroid function=improved fertility) Favorite Brands: Vital Nutrients and Pure Encapsulations
IRON	Helps with fatigue and blood building, specifically anemia. Typically, not recommended to people who are not able to bleed (such as menstruation) as it can build up and cause oxidative damage, however, most women become anemic or close to it at some point in their pregnancy. A lot of people cringe at the thought of taking iron due to its negative effect on digestion, however, if you take a highly absorbable, non-constipating form, you will find that it does not have the same effect. Favorite brands: Biogenesis Ultrahemantic, Thorne Ferrasorb
GLUCOSAMINE	If used in the appropriate dosage and a quality brand, this nutrient does help build cartilage and therefore can decrease joint pain. Favorite Brands: I don't really have a favorite brand for this one. Find one that works for you that is in capsule form.

FENUGREEK	A fantastic fiber and digestive aid, it is also an amazing herb which helps with milk supply during nursing. Favorite Brand: NutriGold

(Professional Monographs, n.d.)

(Hudson, 2008)

RECOMMENDATIONS:

Pre-Conception

1. Prenatal—take what is recommended on the bottle
2. Omega 3—take equivalent to 900-1200mg of EPA (check the back of the bottle, they should break down the omega 3 into EPA and DHA). Try to find a brand and bottle that gives you about 450mg of EPA per capsule.
3. B complex—one capsule daily should suffice, I usually recommend a B50 or B100 if you don't use one of the brands I listed.
4. Vitamin C—1000mg twice daily
5. Vitamin D—a bare minimum of 2000IU but if you live in the northern half of the US, your minimum is likely 5000IU. It is a good idea to get blood levels checked once mid-summer and once deep winter so you know where you are at and can gauge how well you are able to hold onto this fat-soluble vitamin.

6. Calcium/Magnesium—ideally you will take 500mg of calcium twice a day and your complex should complement that with 250-300mg of magnesium twice a day. Check your bottle and make sure you are taking the right amount.
7. Folate (NOT FOLIC ACID!!)—3mg of additional folate. There should be 800-1000mcg in your prenatal.
8. Probiotics—as outlined above, a minimum of 10 billion organisms per capsule. I prefer higher but do what you can.
9. Vitex—750mg one to two times per day to help you get pregnant
10. Rhodiola—200mg daily
11. Vitamin E—400IU daily

First Trimester

1. Prenatal—take what is recommended on the bottle
2. Omega 3-- take equivalent to 1200-1500mg of EPA (check the back of the bottle, they should break down the omega 3 into EPA and DHA). Try to find a brand and bottle that gives you about 450mg of EPA per capsule and take 2 twice daily.
3. Vitamin C—1000mg twice daily to keep your immune system strong. You don't want to get sick during this precious time!
4. Vitamin D—2000IU to 5000IU (or work with your doctor, you may need more)

5. Calcium/Magnesium—ideally you will take 500mg of calcium twice a day and your complex should complement that with 250-300mg of magnesium twice a day. Check your bottle and make sure you are taking the right amount.
6. Folate (NOT FOLIC ACID!!) —3mg to 5mg of additional folate. There should be about 800-1000mcg in your prenatal.
7. Probiotics—as outlined above, a minimum of 10 billion organisms per capsule. I prefer higher but do what you can.

Second Trimester

1. Prenatal—take what is recommended on the bottle
2. Omega 3-- take equivalent to 1200-1500mg of EPA (check the back of the bottle, they should break down the omega 3 into EPA and DHA). Try to find a brand and bottle that gives you about 450mg of EPA per capsule and take 2 twice daily.
3. Vitamin C—1000mg twice daily to keep your immune system strong. You don't want to get sick during this precious time!
4. Vitamin D—2000IU to 5000IU (or work with your doctor, you may need more)
5. Calcium/Magnesium—ideally you will take 500mg of calcium twice a day and your complex should complement that with 250-300mg of magnesium

twice a day. Check your bottle and make sure you are taking the right amount.

6. Folate (NOT FOLIC ACID!!) —3mg to 5mg of additional folate. There should be 800-1000mcg in your prenatal.
7. Probiotics—as outlined above, a minimum of 10 billion organisms per capsule. I prefer higher but do what you can.
8. Iron—you are likely feeling fatigued and may have been told you are anemic. You should take at least one capsule for fatigue but if you have been diagnosed with anemia, increase to 2-3 capsules at bedtime. Dose per capsule is usually between 19-29mg of absorbable iron.
9. Glucosamine—you may begin to have joint pain now and this will help build your connective tissue. I usually recommend about half the dose I would if you were not pregnant so probably 500-1000mg is fine.

Third Trimester

1. Prenatal—take what is recommended on the bottle
2. Omega 3-- take equivalent to 1200-1500mg of EPA (check the back of the bottle, they should break down the omega 3 into EPA and DHA). Try to find a brand and bottle that gives you about 450mg of EPA per capsule and take 2 twice daily.

3. Vitamin C— decrease to 500mg once daily (to prevent possible rebound scurvy when baby is born)
4. Vitamin D—2000IU to 5000IU (or work with your doctor, you may need more)
5. Calcium/Magnesium—ideally you will take 500mg of calcium twice a day and your complex should complement that with 250-300mg of magnesium twice a day. Check your bottle and make sure you are taking the right amount.
6. Folate (NOT FOLIC ACID!!) —3mg is fine
7. Probiotics—as outlined above, a minimum of 10 billion organisms per capsule. I prefer higher but do what you can.
8. Iron—you are likely feeling fatigued and may have been told you are anemic. You should take at least one capsule for fatigue but if you have been diagnosed with anemia, increase to 2-3 capsules at bedtime. Dose per capsule is usually between 19-29mg of absorbable iron.
9. Glucosamine—you may begin to have joint pain now and this will help build your connective tissue. I usually recommend about half the dose I would if you were not pregnant so probably 500-1000mg is fine.
10. Add DHA 1000 from Nordic Naturals: its "game time" for brain development! Take at least two per day in addition to your other omega 3.
11. Add Vitamin E 400IU to help prevent pre-eclampsia (or 400IU every other day).

Breast Feeding

1. Same as 3rd trimester, minus vitamin E and iron
2. Consider upping your DHA 1000 to 3-4 softgels if you really want to go for it!
3. Add Fenugreek—there is nothing better than Fenugreek to help with milk supply. Take about 1500mg 3x per day. I absolutely love the brand NutriGold and recommend it to all of my patients, friends and family.

SECTION 3

"MIXING THE BATTER"

This section is about bringing together all the "goods" to make a perfect baby. A lot of this includes what you have already read but I am going to discuss some genetics as well. The majority of what has already been discussed is absolutely in your control but genetics of course is not. Getting your partner on board is somewhat in your control but only to an extent going by the old saying, "you can lead a horse to water but you can't make him drink". Hopefully he will be as passionate about perfect baby making as you. Perhaps if you tell him that in the long run, there may be less crying, fighting, illness, et cetera but who knows...sometimes people have all the knowledge but still choose a different path.

It is ideal that you both fine tune your diet together, take vitamins together, start to change your lifestyle if you tend to party, start exercising together if you don't already. Make your eggs healthy and make his sperm healthy to give your baby the best possible chance to get optimal DNA that will become his or her genetic make up for life. There are some genetic mishaps you can't change but you can certainly attempt to control them. I am not a geneticist and I would have to write a tremendous amount of material on this extremely confusing topic to help you understand an inkling of what "mixing the batter" REALLY means from a genetic perspective. It is so complicated that it leaves heads spinning in even the most intelligent of people. What I would recommend is that both parents, order a genetic profile online and having it interpreted. You can do this for about $200 each with the 23&Me profile and may be very worth your while and finances. Consider it your first financial drop in the bucket for your baby! The bright side is that you only have to do it once so if you are having more than one baby, this part will already be done. The benefit of doing this type of test is that if you are both carriers of certain diseases, you can predict the chances that your baby will actually HAVE the disease. If you know this, you can be ready if it happens or plan to manage it if it does. There are some genetic issues that cause repeat miscarriages and this could give you peace of mind to know that there is a reason your baby is not making it in the womb—that he or she is structurally not sound or properly equipped to thrive in our big world. More than 50% of miscarriages are due to chromosomal abnormalities. Most of the chromosomal mishaps are due to "poor mixing of the batter" and occur just by chance as the two DNA from mom & dad come together in error. Hopefully, you will read the earlier sections in this book and decrease the chance of THIS sort of mutation from occurring. There are some miscarriages, however, that occur due to genetic defects that are already there, especially if mom has one and dad has one, now baby likely has two.

Chromosomal abnormalities come if various forms of DNA issues: missing pieces, too many pieces, upside down pieces, misplaced pieces or mutated pieces. These genetic material mix-ups are often not life sustaining or they cause severe physical deformities or mental handicaps. Genetic testing is common at around week 13 of pregnancy, especially if you are older parents. Many people opt not to test because they won't terminate regardless of the results so they figure it to be pointless. As you have read, I believe knowledge is power and knowing ahead of time allows you to do research and be prepared ahead of time rather than in the moment of shock. Doing the genetic profile before you even GET pregnant is a great way to be ahead of the game as you may be able to improve your health in relation to some genetic defects that will prevent miscarriage or defects simply by *managing* your genetics.

(Genetic Causes of Female Infertility, n.d.)

The top genetic defect I am referring to is the MTHFR gene. It is strongly associated with fertility and miscarriage as well as spina bifida. MTHFR, the acronym for Methylene TetraHydrofolate Reductase, is an enzyme that is required to convert folate to the active form that can be used by the body. There are several potential mutations in this enzyme that inhibit this ability and therefore put your body at a deficit and put you at risk for a plethora of possible illnesses including heart disease, high cholesterol and blood pressure, Alzheimer's, cancer, stroke, glaucoma and many others. If you recall in the supplement section, I mentioned that I would discuss this supplement more in detail in this section. The reason is that folate helps with spina bifida as it is a required nutrient for closure of the neural tube (basically the spine) and without it, your baby is at high risk of developing spina bifida or on the flip side, high risk of not developing a closed spine and worse, not developing a brain or skull. The problem with the MTHFR mutation is that depending on what type you have, you can take a ton of "folic acid" but it is not the correct form and therefore, it does not protect you or your baby. You must take the active form which comes in few different names: Quatrefolic (R-TM), L-5-MTHF, (6S)-5-Methyltetrahydrofolate. Not everyone does well with all forms and your requirements can vary depending on which mutation you have so it is best to have this tested so that you know what you have. You can then find a practitioner with experience in this field that can help you. There is a website from Dr. Ben Lynch who is the leading expert on MTHFR and taught me everything I know. He has a plethora of research on this and how it is associated with disease and more importantly to you at this current time, your fertility and your baby. Under his "Research" tab, you will find several key research links for various topics. What I have offered here is a baseline knowledge. I recommend that you do your own additional research to expand you own knowledge for your own health, the health of your family and your friends as well.

When I review labs with a patient who has a mutation, I educate that now that we know he/she has the mutation, we can treat the mutation with supplementation. This allows us to bypass the enzyme step of conversion and give your body what it needs without needing to convert it at all. This turns a scary, permanent condition into a treatable one. And THAT is my takeaway message about the genetic aspect of "Mixing the Batter". You and your partner need to take care of your current DNA by eating well, exercising, sleeping, avoid toxins and taking vitamins thus preventing any additional mutations or gene mutation expressions. Educate yourself on your own genetic makeup and shortcomings (because we all have them!). Find ways to improve your odds through lifestyle or supplementation.

(MTHFR, 2014)   (Lynch, n.d.)

SECTION 4

"LET 'EM BAKE"

Congratulations! You're pregnant! The bun is in the oven and you are sitting back and feeling the joy of growing a human being inside your womb. If you were already pregnant when you picked up this book, I hope you are not feeling too defeated. It is NEVER too late to turn things around in your diet and lifestyle, even if you are already 3rd trimester. Everything you do, every minute of the day can affect your baby so don't toss in the towel and figure your baby is doomed! As you are planning for baby's arrival, I have a few suggestions on things that many people do not think about.

FURNITURE

Most people wait until the 3rd trimester or maybe even after the baby is born to think about the nursery or what furniture you want but let me tell you that this is a very bad idea. The furniture has a plethora of chemicals and needs to off-gas for a good amount of time before you put your baby in the nursery and close the door where he/she will sleep for a good portion of their first couple years of life. This often surprises people but I recommend purchasing your furniture and having it assembled by 20 weeks. That gives the furniture another 20 weeks or so to off gas. Keep the door closed and if you are able, open the window either all the time or a good portion of each day to help the chemicals leave, that is an even more optimal thing to do. It is my belief that this (in addition to the crib mattress) are some of the "unknown" reasons for SIDS.

Here are some of the chemicals in furniture and their deleterious effects:

CHEMICAL	PRIMARY SOURCES	HARMFUL EFFECTS
Volatile Organic Compounds (VOCs)	Paint, lacquer, cleaning supplies, varnish, wax, plywood & particle board (and many other sources)	Irritation of mucous membranes, headaches, nausea, loss of coordination. Damage to multiple organs and also carcinogenic.
Poly-brominated diphenyl ethers (PBDEs)	Plastics, furniture foam, fabrics, et cetera that are treated with flame retardant.	Endocrine/ hormone disruptor, neurological & reproductive damage. Animal studies have shown neurobehavioral and thyroid damage to babies exposed prenatally and through breast milk. Studies also show a link to obesity.
Polyvinyl Chloride	Baby	Linked to breast

(PVC)	mattresses, furniture, upholstery, wall coverings, ceiling tiles, carpet, window treatments plus pipes, conduits, and many other materials.	cancer, decreased fertility, miscarriages, stillborn, decreased sperm count, asthma in children
Perfluorinated compounds (PFC's)	Non-stick cookware (Teflon) Stain resistant fabrics such as on couches and carpet	Affects growth and development and causes low birth weight when exposed prenatally. Affects liver function and reproductive function. Animal studies show delayed growth and development when exposed.
Perchloro-ethylene (PCE)	Dry cleaning Aerosols, furniture polish, lubricant, adhesives	Dizziness and loss of consciousness but long-term exposure can cause cancer, damage to kidneys and liver

		and memory loss.
Antimony Oxide	Flame retardant	Known carcinogen
Formaldehyde	Furniture, particle board (cabinets, flooring, insulation), curtains, soap, detergent and glues. Also used in mattress fabrics.	Mild exposure can cause headaches, insomnia, fatigue and respiratory problems. Directly associated with multiple cancers but leukemia, brain cancer and nasopharyngeal cancer in particular.
Triclosan	Anti-bacterial soap Furniture Toys	Endocrine disruptor
Chlorine	Wood pulp Mold removal	Lung disease Tooth corrosion
Ammonia	Glass cleaners Furniture cleaners	Irritation to mucous membranes and lungs and also lung damage and death at higher levels of exposures.
Xylene	Adhesives in mattresses	Birth defects (confirmed by the EPA)
Toluene Discarnate	Foam in mattresses	Skin irritation and respiratory issues

Benzene	Memory foam	Known carcinogen

(Scutti, 2013) (The Scary Chemicals in Your Sofa, 2012) (Lee, 2013)

(Are Toxins in Your Furniture Making You Sick, 2008)

(Are Toxic Chemicals Lurking in your Furniture and Building Products?, 2010)

(Doward, n.d.)

CRIB MATTRESS

As you can see in the chart listed above, there are many chemicals in general but several are used in mattresses, including your baby mattress. Your baby is laying in his/her crib for 12-17 hours a day, potentially breathing in toxic chemicals. Perhaps this is why the "back to sleep" movement decreased the incidences of SIDS but still 15,000 babies died in 2013 of SIDS world-wide. The highest rate of SIDS is month 2-4 of life which, coincidentally is when parents often transition babies to their crib. This theory was adamantly opposed and claimed to be unfounded in a press release in 1998 against a man named Barry Richardson who felt that SIDS was indeed a result of antimony found in crib mattresses. The opposing press release claims that antimony is not the cause of death and that mattresses are safe. However, one common flame retardant that used to be applied to baby pajamas was made illegal due to findings that it caused DNA mutations and ultimately cancer. That same chemical is still allowed in crib mattresses. The offender is called Tris and is found in most mattresses tested as reported by the Chicago Tribune in an article written in December 2012. A more recent study that was published in the 2014 February issue of Environmental Science and Technology and reported on FoxNews Health in April 2014 found that VOC exposure was extremely high in a baby's sleeping area. In fact, exposure was twice as high inside the crib as it was just outside the crib in the same room. Plus, in addition to the extra hours of sleep, babies breathe in more air per body weight thus increasing exposure by 10-fold compared to adults. The researchers suggested using older mattresses (with caution due to changing regulations in allowable chemicals!) or giving ample time for the mattress to off gas (which is what I am suggesting with the 20-week nursery set up rule). I also suggest using an organic crib mattress pad that has been thoroughly washed and rinsed prior to use.

When it comes to chemicals and their possible detrimental effects and potential link to SIDS, the reality is we just don't know! So, why not err on the side of caution? An organic mattress is about twice the cost of a regular mattress but worth the extra money as your baby will sleep well over 4000 hours on that mattress in the first year alone! Regardless of research, proven or disproven, speculated or confirmed, that is a LOT of time to spend on a mattress so this is not the place to penny pinch. Instead of a fancy diaper bag, use an old backpack instead and throw the extra $100 at the mattress.

(Toxic Gas Hypothesis, 1998) (Hawthorne, 2012)

(Crib Mattresses Release Potentially Harmful Chemicals, study finds, 2014)

DETERGENT, FABRIC SOFTENER, SOAP, LOTION AND MORE

I am lumping these things together because they all have something in common—chemicals that are known to cause cancer, liver damage, neurotoxicity, reproductive toxicity, endocrine disruption and general biochemical disruptions. These chemicals are absorbed into the skin, into YOUR skin and can affect your fertility when you are trying to get pregnant and into your baby if you are already pregnant. If you are nursing, it affects both you and baby. This probably sounds extreme and you may be rolling your eyes, but even drugs are now created because we have learned how easily the skin will absorb chemicals. There is the nicotine patch for one then there are several hormone patches, hormones creams/gels, anti-nausea patches, pain patches, birth control patches, and many, many more pharmaceuticals that use “skin absorption” as a vehicle to change blood chemistry. I had an epiphany several years ago when I was working in the yard doing some serious yardwork in the sun and I was sweating and suddenly I was overwhelmed with the smell of my Victoria’s Secret lotion that I had put on the day before at 6am, after my morning shower. So, here it was, about 30 hours later and the scent was so strong I felt the need to get away from myself and I thought, "oh my goodness...the sun is baking chemicals into my skin!" And that was the day I switched to organic lotion and eventually soap, shampoo, conditioner, sunscreen and stopped wearing perfume except for about twice a year for a VERY special occasion. Everything that comes into contact with our skin, especially for prolonged periods, will be absorbed. Chemicals from laundry detergent and fabric softeners, dryer sheets, deodorants, lotions, soaps, everything! I am not suggesting you become a smelly free bird of course. What I am suggesting, is that during this precious time, you do opt to spend a little more on organic products. It will give you an opportunity to try out different brands and decide if you want to keep them around once baby is older. I would suggest keeping them for baby for much longer though as they are more susceptible to absorbing these chemicals and having them build up in their little bodies. Again, could this be why children are having so many more issues these days? Increases in childhood illnesses and behavioral issues are dramatic. People are scratching their heads at this oddity but look at the chemicals that are everywhere, all the time. We wash our sheets and dry them with dryer sheets then we sleep in them for over a third of our life and kids for even longer while the toxins seep into our blood. We put on clothes laden with chemicals, flush with our skin 24 hours a day, 7 days a week and they absolutely do leak chemicals into our body. In fact, there have been many recalls in clothing, babies and adults alike due to toxic chemicals. To put it in perspective, Alaska Airlines had to replace uniforms for over 32,000 flight attendants because the materials were making people extremely ill, some with rashes, others with immune system debilitation and hormone disruption. The chemicals could not be washed away with laundering and continued to make people sick every time they wore them. Greenpeace has also been investigating the toxic chemicals (phthalates, amines, NPEs and azo dyes in particular) that are known carcinogens and endocrine disruptors as well as causing other health issues.

There is, of course, a huge environmental impact as well but I will let you look that up yourself and I am going to save these pages for their intended topics. I would recommend reading the article by Dr. Mercola, "Are You Poisoning Your Household With this Chore?" as it is fantastically useful in understanding the big picture.

(Highly toxic chemicals are found in laundry detergents, dryer sheets, deodorants, perfumes, soaps and other household products, 2004)

(Mercola, Are You Poisoning Your Household With this Chore?, 2011)

(Tide Detergent Found To Contain High Levels Of 1,4-Dioxane, Carcinogenic Contaminant, 2012)

(Cancer Jean Risk, 2014)

(Alaska Air replaces uniforms after attendants say it sickened them, 2013)

(Big Fashion Stitch Up, 2012) (Toxic Recalls and Recall Information)

In summary, do the best you can to limit known chemicals in your furniture, your baby's furniture, your personal products, your cleaning products and your house in general. During this precious time, limit exposure to "new things" as much as possible. If you have no choice, try to let things off gas outside your home or in your garage before bringing them inside if at all possible. When baby is born, wash everything, twice, in organic detergent and dry with chemical free dryer sheets (BabyGanics makes a great one!). Remember it is impossible to live in a chemical-free world but you can use your new knowledge to be picky for the sake of your fertility, your unborn baby and your born baby's future. So, as you enjoy your pregnancy and bond with your baby through all of his/her movements inside you and contemplate your life with your newborn, continue to educate yourself on the best ways to support your baby, his/her future, your bond, your marriage and your new life.

SECTION 5

"THE COOLING PHASE"

The baby is born! You are finally holding your tiny treasure. YOU created this masterpiece! It is out of the oven and your life will never be the same again. You now know a love that only a parent can know. Everyone can tell you but you don't really know it until you have felt it yourself. It is the most beautiful, painful, exhilarating, tortuous, glorious feeling in the world! You've made it this far. You're about 2/3 of the way done and now you have a whole additional year to nourish your baby THROUGH you with good food, good habits, good air, a positive and loving environment and many other aspects of your life. This is where I am going to take the opportunity to discuss breast feeding.

You can tell by the previous content that I am pro-breast feeding. I believe with all my heart that it is the best gift you can give to your child that will last a lifetime. The 6-12 months prior to conception is ideal, during pregnancy is required but then a good portion of people just give up after that and default to "what's easy" because they are tired of the sacrifice. But ladies, MOMMIES! Hear me out please! This is the greatest sacrifice you can give and it is just 12 more months of your life. And if this is one of two babies or the only baby you plan on having, why not?? If you are having more, then it ups the ante, doesn't it? But no need to shortchange the younger babies on behalf of the older kids. Each child should be a 2-3-year journey and breast feeding, in my opinion, should be a non-negotiable part of that journey if you are able to do it. If you were on a trip from California to Maine and you got to Illinois ran out of gas and were too tired to go on, would you quit? No! You would get a hotel, get rested, fuel up your car and keep going. If you were running a marathon and hit the proverbial wall at mile 18, wouldn't you keep going until you crossed the finish line? Of course! You've come this far, so complete your mission!

All the breast-feeding experts will tell you how amazing it is and how natural it is and although it is natural, it is HARD in the beginning. A challenge for so many reasons and a struggle to believe in your own body. Believe that it WILL make enough milk to nourish your baby and that your baby will learn how to do it and survive. Believe that the pain will eventually decrease and that you two will eventually get into a groove and you will both figure it out. I will tell you that it can take up to *three months* to really establish your milk supply. And you may need to give a little supplemental formula here and there but try to relax and know that with patience and time, the glorious nectar will flow freely for your baby. And when you can nurse and sleep and barely notice that your baby was awake 3 times in the night, you will be so grateful. And when baby is having a meltdown and you can just pull off the road and climb in the back seat and not worry about the perfect temperature water and mixing and shaking formula, you will be so grateful. And when your baby gets older and doesn't get as sick as the other kids or have as many health or behavioral issues, you can pat yourself on the back and figure it was all because you gave this sacrifice for 12 short months.

There was a day in the early part of the 20th century and into the 1970's that doctors recommended mothers NOT breastfeed and about 80% of mothers had their babies on the bottle (formula) at that time. Since then, we have slowly learned all of the health benefits of breast feeding and it is now on the rise again with about 75% of mothers' breast feeding for at least a portion of time, the majority (44.4%) breast feeding to 6 months and less than a fourth (23.4%) lasting to one year. The Surgeon General, CDC, Mayo Clinic, World Health Organization and many more experts all recommend nursing for at least 12 months for optimal health. And new research published in the NIH from the Journal of Perinatal Education, came out that showed formula is linked to diabetes, obesity, eczema, asthma and allergies as well as many other illnesses. They also found that the longer children were breastfed, the more protection they had from these diseases and illnesses.

(Fischer, 2011)

(Breast feeding rate has increased but few mothers are nursing for the recommended time, 2013)

(Emily E Stevens, 2009, Spring)

BENEFITS OF BREAST FEEDING

Here are the many benefits of breast feeding broken down for you:

FOR BABY:

1. Decreases/prevents illnesses such as ear infections, pneumonia and diarrhea
2. Decreases incidence of asthma, allergies and eczema
3. Decrease risk of obesity
4. Decreases risk of diabetes, both type 1 and type 2
5. Decreases risk of Celiac Disease
6. Reduces risk of Sudden Infant Death Syndrome (SIDS)
7. Decreases risk of leukemia
8. Less colic due to less digestive upset and improved gut flora for life
9. Helps with brain development and is associated with higher IQ later in life
10. Less crying as it is quicker to meet baby's needs, especially at night

FOR MOM

1. Decreases incidence of breast, endometrial and ovarian cancer

2. Decreases incidence of Type 2 diabetes
3. Easier time losing weight—breast feeding burns between 500-700 calories per day (that's like running 5-7 miles!!)
4. Reduces post-partum depression
5. Due to oxytocin release, helps decrease chance of post-partum hemorrhage and helps the uterus recover more quickly
6. Decreases risk of anemia after pregnancy
7. Decreased chance of pregnancy while nursing (and usually no periods for at least 6 months!)
8. Decreases risk of osteoporosis later in life

OTHER BENEFITS

1. Saves $1200-$1500 in formula expenses
2. Improves the bond between mom and baby due to skin to skin contact and forced down time with baby
3. Readily available anytime, anywhere
4. Changes to adapt to growing baby's needs and even changes during the day with more water in the morning milk and more fat in the nighttime milk.
5. Globally, less healthcare costs and 800,000 less infant deaths per year

(Breastfeeding Fact Sheet, 2011) (Breastfeeding benefits, 2014)

(10 Facts on Breastfeeding , 2015) (Church, 2013)

I would assume or at least hope that I have convinced you enough with all the listed benefits. I would encourage you to talk to your partner and get him on board, or hopefully he is reading this book with you. He needs to support your decision to breast feed otherwise you may default to what is easy rather than what is best for your baby.

Of course, there are some instances that breast feeding just doesn't work for you anymore or you cannot endure the stress of trying to build your milk supply despite drinking a gallon of water per day and taking the fenugreek as suggested in the supplement section. Be kind to yourself and know that formula has come a long way and now has a ton of omega 3 fatty acids and that your baby will be just fine either way. My one suggestion here is that IF you decide to add in formula or if you must add in formula to supplement, get an organic formula and consider using the sensitive tummy version. My favorite brand is Earth's Best and I have found that babies tolerate the sensitive version better than the regular version.

DIAPERS

Oh yes, the diaper dilemma! If you are one of the great parents that will do cloth diapers, I commend you. Be sure you are using that special detergent though so that means no diaper service unless they guarantee they are not using bleach and that they are using a low or no-chemical detergent, otherwise, it's not much better for baby or the environment. There will be a time that you will need to use disposable diapers for traveling or outings so this information is still relevant. If you are one of the dads or moms (like me) that can't stomach the thought of cloth diapers or don't want to put that on your caregiver, then this becomes an extremely important section for you to read and implement. Babies are in diapers for an average of 900 to 1200 days (some more, some less). That is a total of about 22,000 to nearly 30,000 hours with their bottoms cover by a diaper so based on what we have gone over so far, you now KNOW they will be absorbing chemicals and in a very precious place no less!

The two main chemicals in conventional diapers are dioxin and sodium polyacrylate. These chemicals are known to cause a plethora of health issues including cancer, multiple organ damage, endocrine & hormone disruption, reproductive damage, immune suppression, diabetes, respiratory problems (including asthma) and allergic reactions. Some diapers contain a number of other chemicals which are known to cause obesity, arrhythmia, cancer, neurotoxicity, lung & kidney damage and other potential issues as minor as a rash and as severe as death. These are, of course, at extreme levels of exposure but I feel it is in your baby's best interest to try to keep these out of your baby's life for as long as possible. Livestrong reported on a study published in 1999 in the Archives of Environmental Health that claimed the chemicals in disposable diapers may be the cause of the rise in asthma in children over recent years. Even if I told you there was 5% chance your child could get one of these illnesses and you knew you could prevent it, wouldn't you? And we don't actually know what the chances are so it's best to not take any chances since there are fantastic alternatives out there.

(The Harmful Chemicals in Disposable Diapers, 2012)

(Kassem, 2013)   (Sharratt, 2010)

You will have to go by trial and error so try not to buy mass quantities of any one brand until you know you love it. My absolute favorite is Bambo Nature and some of my other top choices are BabyGanics, Earth's Best and Seventh Generation. I loved Naty with my daughter but they did not work for my son, so, again, you will need to try different types and see what works best based on your baby and based on your lifestyle. Every year these natural diapers seem to improve so you are blessed that there are companies out there that have figured it out! Be sure to share your choices with your friends and family so you don't get saturated with conventional diapers at your baby shower! I suggest putting the diapers you want to try directly on your baby registry so that people know you are going natural. When baby starts sleeping through the night, you may become tempted to use the overnight types from those other brands. I suggest trying a diaper that is the next size up and diapering up to the belly button to increase coverage.

AIR FRESHENERS

I figured that a discussion about air fresheners is perfectly placed after diapers. Diaper pails are smelly, no matter what kind of diapers you use. And people usually don't want their homes to smelly like poopy diapers. As a result, many, many people turn to chemical air fresheners such as plug-ins or various things in that category. Before I even begin to tell you about the chemicals in these things, I must say, do NOT put these things in your baby's room, or your room for that matter. Breathing those things for hours on end will harm you in some way. The chemicals found in air fresheners are similar to many we have already discussed with the same detrimental effects of course. The Natural Resources Defense Council tested several different air fresheners and over 85% of them had phthalates. As discussed earlier, phthalates are known to be an endocrine disruptor which means they cause hormonal abnormalities, reproductive/fertility problems and birth defects. Air fresheners also contain VOCs, benzene and formaldehyde which all have an array of detrimental health issues including abnormal development of male genitalia (when exposed in utero), increased asthma, low testosterone, decrease in sperm quality and other issues, most of which we have already discussed. Care2 Healthy Living reported on an article from MSN that claimed asthma incidence can be increased by as much as 71% when exposed to air fresheners.

You may be thinking, well fine, I will just burn candles then (I know, I thought the same thing!) but unfortunately, they are toxic too. Despite being banned by the EPA in 2003, lead wicks are still found in 30% of candles sold in America. If they are made outside of the US, they likely have a lead wick. Inhalation exposure to the burning lead has been linked to hormone disruption, asthma, learning disabilities, et cetera. Even if the candles have regular wicks, the chemicals in the burning wax can be as bad as if you were smoking cigarettes indoors with the windows closed or breathing exhaust from the back of a car. Candles contain paraffin which when burned and inhaled has been linked to cancer of the liver and kidneys in lab rats. And most candles contain benzene, ketones and toluene which are harmful for a number of reasons but have been linked to asthma and have been found to induce an asthma attack. Time Magazine published an article in 2009 that said researchers have found a link between asthma and lung cancer to burning candles indoors.

So, although this new knowledge falls in the post-delivery section, this should be a lifelong change for your whole family. Basically, no air fresheners and no commercial candles. Beeswax and soybean candles are technically safe. Essential oils in water under a beeswax tea light in a proper set up (Try Bath and Body Works or The Body Shop) are great as well.

(Toxic Air Fresheners, 2011)

(Exposed: Cancer-Causing Toxins Found in Air Fresheners, 2012)

(Avoid Harsh Chemicals in Commercial Air Fresheners with Homemade Alternatives, 2012)

(Toxins in Candles: Sad but True) (Are Your Candles Toxic?, 2014)

(Don't use scented candles, n.d.) (Blue, 2009)

(Can burning candles make you sick? University studies scrutinize possible release of toxic fumes, 201)

BABY PRODUCTS

VASELINE/BABY OIL

I have covered the chemicals and dangers of products we put on our skin in detail thus far. People make the gross generalization that if it is made for baby then it is safe for baby. This is tragically an inaccurate assumption. Many baby products (some are handed out in the hospital!), have petroleum products in them such as Vaseline, baby oil, mineral oil, etc. Petroleum comes from crude oil and is a waste product when making gasoline. It is purified (of course), otherwise, it would not be white but there may be some of the polyaromatic hydrocarbons (PAH) left behind that are known carcinogens and endocrine disruptors. Not to mention, the body recognizes it as a toxin so when it gets into our body it builds up and causes acne, cancer, reproductive problems, developmental delays, neurotoxicity and organ damage. The skin is not only our largest organ but it is also our largest organ of detoxification so when you apply petroleum products to the skin, it prevents exit of toxins the body may be trying to get rid of, no entry, no exit. It has been banned by the European Union and restricted in Canada so although America still considers it "safe", perhaps it is not. It is best to use an organic or petroleum free equivalent such as Baby Bee (Burt's Bees) Multipurpose ointment or Earth Mama Angel Baby Bottom Balm or Babyganics Protective Ointment. For oils, there are lots of people who use organic coconut oil topically. Or you can buy baby specific option such as California Baby's oil or a good lotion from Burt's Bee Baby Bee.

(Petroleum jelly - Identification, toxicity, use, water pollution potential, ecological toxicity and regulatory information)

(What's Wrong with Vaseline?, 2013)

(Petrolum Health Concerns)

(Harmful Toxic Toiletries)

BABY POWDER

In addition to petroleum, talc is used in baby powder and is known to cause respiratory problems (and lung cancer) and has been linked to ovarian cancer and endometrial cancer when used in the pelvic area. For obvious reasons, baby powder is not recommended unless you buy talc-free baby powder. JASON's brand makes one as well as California Baby and Nature's baby.

(Talcum Powder and Cancer, 2014)

(Horowitz, 2000) (Talcum Powder Linked to Ovarian Cancer, 2008)

WIPES

If diapers, oils, lotions are not bad enough, there is a long list of chemicals in baby wipes as well (of course!). Most fall into the same categories we have already discussed but a new one I came across is called Methylisothiazolinone (MI) and has been linked to severe rashes in children with use of wipes containing this ingredient. There are other ingredients as well such as Disodium EDTA, PEG-40, Trisodium Citrate, Phenoyethanol, Ehtyhyxylgylcerin, Benzyl Alcohol, Sodium Benzoate, BIS-PEG/PPG-16, Dimethicone and "Fragrance" (catch-all for lots of chemicals). That is a long list of chemicals that you will be wiping over your baby's bum and probably neck when they are nursing and hands and face when they are older. Try an organic/natural brand like Naty, Earth's Best, Babyganics or something similar. They still have a few chemicals but way less and some of them use organic ingredients, non-GMO, no artificial flavors, colors or preservatives, etc. Alternatively, you can use a wash cloth and water when you are home and there is a new brand of wipes called WaterWipes that are genuinely just water based. So do your research and don't slather your baby's body with something you would panic if they were eating it.

(Baby Wipe Chemical Tied to Allergic Reactions in Some Kids, 2014)

(INNES, 2014)

OTHER POTENTIAL CHEMICALS IN BABY PRODUCTS

CHEMICAL	**TYPICAL PRODUCTS**	**ADVERSE EFFECTS**
Ceteareth (Chemicals to Avoid in Baby Care Products)	Bath products Sunscreen Lotion	Neurotoxicity Organ damage Skin rashes
DEET (Seems to be controversial)	Bug sprays	Organ damage Reproductive damage

(Adams, 2004) (Diep, 2014) (DEET, 2014) (Dangers of DEET, 2014) (Is it true that the DEET used in most mosquito repellents is toxic? , 2008) (Chemicals to Avoid in Baby Care Products)		Causes DNA mutations Neurological damage Seizures Rashes Death
Dimethyl phthalate (DMP) (Chemicals to Avoid in Baby Care Products) (Hazardous Substance Fact Sheet: Dimethyl phthalate) (Dimethyl Phthalate, 2000)	Baby insect repellent	Immune toxicity Respiratory toxicity Damage to liver/kidneys Carcinogenic (cancer) Teratogenic Endocrine/ Hormone disruptor
Octinoxate (Octinoxate: uses, benefits and dangers) (Loux, 2012)	Sunscreen	Endocrine/ Hormone disruptor Increases estrogen & may be linked to

(Chemicals to Avoid in Baby Care Products)		breast cancer Decreases thyroid hormones Low sperm count
Oxybenzone (Loux, 2012)	Sunscreen	Endocrine/ Hormone disruptor Skin rash/eczema
Octocrylene (Loux, 2012)	Sunscreen	DNA mutation Cell damage
Homosalate (Loux, 2012)	Sunscreen	Endocrine/ Hormone disruptor
Butylparaben Ethylparaben Methylparaben Propylparaben (Loux, 2012) (Adams K.)	Sunscreen	Endocrine/ Hormone disruptor Reproductive damage Developmental toxicity Possible link to breast cancer
PABA (Wittman, 2015) (Chemicals to Avoid in Baby Care Products)	Sunscreen Lotion	DNA damage Hormone disruptor Allergic reactions Liver Damage Skin damage/skin cancer

<u>Phthalates</u> **See previous sections (Chemicals to Avoid in Baby Care Products) (Phthalates: Harmful Effects of the Agent, 2003)	Anything with the word "Fragrance" including lotions, baby bath, baby shampoos et cetera	Liver failure Kidney Failure Endocrine/ Hormone disruptor Lung irritant & damage
<u>Triclosan</u> (Chemicals to Avoid in Baby Care Products) (Glaser) (FDA: Triclosan: What Consumers Should Know, 2013) (Steckelberg, 2014)	Baby soap Baby shampoo Anti-bacterial soap	Endocrine/ Hormone disruptor Immune System contaminant Reproductive damage Cancer (linked to dioxins)
<u>Triethanolamine (TEA)</u> (Chemicals to Avoid in Baby Care Products) (Triethanolamine) (Triethanolamine)	Fragrance in various products	Immune system disruptor Respiratory damage Skin rash/damage Organ damage Liver cancer Bladder cancer Testicular cancer

In summary, there are so many chemicals in baby products that could potentially harm your baby both in the short term and in the long term. The best option is to stay away from conventional products and stick to organic-based baby products. Nothing is going to be perfect but it will be significantly less harmful to your baby. It is worth the time to do a little research and worth the extra money to buy higher quality, less chemical infused products. They last a long time anyway (I used the same tube of diaper cream for over a year so who cares if it is $7 instead of $3, right?). It goes to the short-term pain for long term gain theory. Again, if you are registering for baby products, it would be a good idea to only register for products you are willing to use so you don't have to donate everything, return everything or be tempted to use it "because you have it".

SECTION 6

"THE FROSTING ON THE CAKE—ENJOYING THE FINISHED PRODUCT"

You have your baby home, you're nursing, and you're getting into your groove. Now is not the time to deprioritize everything you have learned. In some ways, babies are MORE susceptible to the choices you make during the first year. You may have been able to get away with the occasional coffee while pregnant but now your baby protests. You were probably able to eat broccoli during pregnancy but now baby gets gassy and uncomfortable. There are some things we can ingest or intake freely during pregnancy but that now harm baby or cause discomfort through nursing. This is not a reason to give up nursing, it is just a reminder that the 2-year journey of sacrifice is not over.

This is the "frosting" on your baby cake! Cake is great but cake with frosting is way better, right? So, keep up the good work! You are almost free to return to your vices should you choose to go that route. For now, you should be doing all of the following things:

1. Taking your vitamins! See the earlier supplement section but I want to reiterate that DHA is a MUST have at this point. Give your baby brain food to help him/her grow. Just to re-iterate, studies show that DHA supplementation improves brain development, increases IQ,

improves communication and social development, and improves sensory development and motor development.

2. Exercising daily—you DO have time! Put the baby in the stroller or in the baby carrier and at least go for a walk. Take turns with your husband going to the gym. Switch off with another mom—she watches your kid for an hour, you watch her kid for an hour. Find a way to start back as soon as you are released from your doctor to do so (usually 1-2 weeks for vaginal delivery and 5-6 weeks for caesarean)
3. Using natural/organic diapers and wipes
4. Using natural/organic baby products including diaper cream, lotion, baby shampoo, baby soap, talc-free powder, oils, sunscreen, et cetera
5. Washing your new clothes and baby's new clothes before wearing
6. Using natural/organic laundry detergent for you and baby (baby is ON you a lot in the first few months so your clothes matter too! I washed all my nursing shirts and tanks with my baby's clothes to be safe)
7. Continuing to eat a relatively clean, whole foods diet
8. Avoiding alcohol & caffeine
9. DO NOT resuming smoking (or other drugs) if you quit

10. Now is the time to communicate with your spouse when you will resume intimacy and check in with him to make sure both of you are feeling supported in the division of duties.
11. Start to make a plan of how your life will be if you are returning to work.
12. Do not buy too many "new things" without letting them off-gas first, ideally in the garage or somewhere away from where baby is spending most of his/her time.
13. Enjoy every minute with your baby, the good and the bad.
14. Snuggle with your baby as much as possible.
15. Take hundreds of pictures and video to show off your masterpiece!

If this list seems daunting, remember, you are at mile 20 of a marathon and sometimes the last 6.2 are the hardest because you know you are almost there but it seems like it is taking forever. I can assure you though that you WILL cross the finish line and on your baby's first birthday, when he/she is enjoying their little mini organic carrot cake for the first time with a beeswax candle in the center, you can sit back and revel in your glory!

FOOD INTRODUCTION

As cute as it may seem to watch your baby eat, I strongly discourage food introduction at all prior to 6 months of age. Early food introduction puts baby at risk of developing food allergies. People often think you have to start with a baby cereal but that is not correct. Your baby may be excited to eat as he/she has seen you do over and over so baby will be thrilled to finally experience something new in his or her mouth. Their little faces tend to tell a different story but they usually come back for more. In general, here are my recommendations for food introduction and the first 6 months of food eating (ages 6-12 months):

1. No sooner than 6 months (or 24 weeks of age at the earliest)
2. Start with a single ingredient food. I started with rice cereal mixed with breast milk for both of my kids followed by oatmeal. Some people start with yams mixed with breast milk or protein/meat mixed with breast milk.
3. Use only your own homemade food or an organic brand that does not use GMO ingredients. I prefer Earth's Best, Plum Organics and Happy Family Organics.
4. Introduce one new food every 3 days so that if baby has a reaction, you know which food is responsible.
5. Do not introduce dairy until one year of age or older (if at all) and stick with good quality organic cheese and organic yogurt as a source of dairy (not milk).
6. Avoid any sugar based products until one year of age or older.

7. Do not give them juice, never, ever, ever! This is such a waste of calories and just pure sugar and sets them up to dislike water.
8. Only give them water and put it everywhere once they have the ability to use a sippy cup. I bought the Green Sprouts glass (with plastic sleeve) sippy cups or the Fogo sippy cups and put two around the house and both of my kids LOVE water and refuse juice and they drink in in quantities that would put most adults to shame. They (like you) need half of their body weight in ounces (meaning a 30-pound baby needs 15 ounces of water per day).
9. Once they have a few teeth, start giving them soft beans like black beans or pinto beans. They love to pick up these little treasures with their new found fine motor skills and put them in their mouth.
10. Never, ever give them white bread. I started my kids on Dave's Killer Bread and that is all they know. My daughter had white bread for the first time when she was about 5 years old and she came home and said, "Mommy, I had the most amazing bread! It was so soft and almost melted in my mouth!" I asked if it was white and she said "Yes!" then I burst out laughing and explained she would have to enjoy that at her friend's house because it would never enter our home. I occasionally buy the softer breads but they are still organic of course. You could even try gluten-free bread if you want although it lacks

protein and fiber and therefore defeats the purpose in my opinion.

11. Just like the advice I give in the Basic Food Tips, avoid white food with the children as well. Once they get a taste for it, it is hard to go back. Use yams instead of potatoes, give them brown rice instead of white (later of course) or quinoa and don't feel like pasta is your only go to for food. In fact, we have pasta about once a year in my house. It is not a staple at all but bean burritos definitely are a quick go-to and filled with guacamole, pico and organic refried black beans. The baby gets the beans and guacamole for now.
12. Try lentils and green chickpeas, hummus, organic edamame (limited) and homemade soups. You will be surprised what the babies will eat...probably even healthier than you can at times!

This is a precious time to introduce things and if you do it right and stand firm even when there are more convenient options, your baby will develop a palate for healthier things because he or she won't KNOW the other things. How could you say cheesecake is your favorite thing if you had never had it?

BOTTLES AND SIPPY CUPS

There are a plethora of bottles and sippy cups that are made from plastic and they are so cute with their bright colors and gender specific themes. Don't be fooled though, they are filled with xenoestrogens just like all the other plastics. They may be BPA free but there are plenty of other chemicals that feature the same hormone disrupting properties that we just haven't discovered yet or that has not been released to the public. When it comes to nursing and pumping, there are not many options out there. I recommend pumping into Medela bottles and transferring it to the nursing bags and freezing as soon as possible. If you plan to use the milk within the appropriate window of freshness, I recommend transferring it to the glass bottle you plan to feed baby in. Same goes for formula if you end up going that route, use glass bottles primarily. Your baby will have his or her favorite so it is best to buy 1-2 of several brands and see which one baby gravitates towards (or doesn't leak all over!). We successfully used Life Factory and Evenflo glass bottles. Additional options include BornFree, Philips AVENT, Dr. Brown's, which all make glass bottles. For sippy cups, we used Fogo, LifeFactory and the Green Sprouts with the glass insert which I mentioned before.

FORMULA

As I have discussed, breastmilk is the best milk for your baby but there may be reasons out of your control that you cannot breastfeed or there may be logistical complications that prevent you from breastfeeding. If you are struggling or just really can't do it, the experts say if you can try to make it to 3 months, it will give your baby less of a chance of developing diabetes and other complications associated with early introduction of cow's milk proteins. When it comes time, you are then forced to make a choice about the best formula for your baby. As I mentioned earlier in the book, I recommend Earth's Best Sensitive Formula and I also like the Vermont Organics. As soon as my baby turned one, I discovered Kabrita Goat milk formula and switched to decrease his exposure to cow's milk. If I would have found this sooner, I probably would have started him at 10 months.

A NOTE ON VACCINES

Vaccines are an integral part of the first year of life (and beyond). This is such a controversial topic and I have chosen to leave it out of this book intentionally. I encourage you to educate yourself and do what you feel is best for your baby and for your family. If you choose to vaccinate according to the CDC schedule, my recommendation is that you find a physician that knows how to boost or modulate your baby's immune system to protect them as much as possible (such as probiotics and methylfolate). If you want to vaccinate but want to follow a modified schedule, find a physician that will work with you on creating an alternative. If you choose not to vaccinate, be sure to take extra precautions with your baby as to not expose him or her to anything that you would not want them to endure and also protect others if you suspect he or she was exposed. For further information, I recommend reading through the CDC guidelines (found online) and then doing multiple searches on the internet regarding pros and cons of vaccines, adverse effects, pros and cons of a modified schedule, etc. And of course, be sure you and your partner are aligned in your approach.

CONCLUSION

Congratulations! Your perfect or almost perfect baby was created because you and your partner made a choice to devote two years of your life to clean-living. There is no greater gift you can give your baby. Now move forward and pick and choose which of these changes you will stick with for yourself and your family. I do encourage you to try to stay on course regarding things your baby is exposed to or consumes because he or she can't choose for at least a decade or more. You will be so thankful you made the choices you made or continue to make as you watch the contrary in other families. These things make a dramatic difference and you will see it for yourself over the years. Again, short term pain for long term gain. Your children will thank you some day!

REFERENCES

http://www.drugs.com/pregnancy-categories.html

http://americanpregnancy.org/medication/medication-and-pregnancy/

http://www.fda.gov/Drugs/DrugSafety/ucm245470.htm

http://www.webmd.com/infertility-and-reproduction/features/infertility-stress

http://www.thyroid.org/thyroid-disease-pregnancy/

http://www.niddk.nih.gov/health-information/health-topics/endocrine/pregnancy-and-thyroid-disease/Pages/fact-sheet.aspx

http://www.niehs.nih.gov/health/topics/agents/endocrine/

http://static.ewg.org/pdf/kab_dirty_dozen_endocrine_disruptors.pdf?_ga=1.208456090.98234801.1446681069

http://www.ncbi.nlm.nih.gov/pmc/articles/PMC2649233/

http://www.natural-health-for-fertility.com/xenoestrogen.html

http://www.natural-health-for-fertility.com/

http://www.babyhopes.com/articles/hormones-conception.html

http://www.womenfitness.net/FSH_role.htm

http://www.whattoexpect.com/pregnancy/pregnancy-health/pregnancy-hormones/estrogen.aspx

http://natural-fertility-info.com/estrogen-fertility-guide.html

http://www.sciencedaily.com/releases/2014/03/140304141948.htm

http://www.webmd.com/women/guide/normal-testosterone-and-estrogen-levels-in-women

https://www.womentowomen.com/adrenal-health-2/dhea-and-adrenal-imbalance/2/

http://www.aicr.org/enews/2014/08-august/faq-processed-meat-and.html

http://www.cbc.ca/news/health/bacon-deli-meat-may-raise-pancreatic-cancer-risk-1.1275319

http://www.today.com/food/5-things-you-need-know-about-deli-meats-2D80554934

http://www.ncbi.nlm.nih.gov/pmc/articles/PMC2967503/

http://www.livestrong.com/article/291530-sodium-nitrate-consumption-during-pregnancy/

http://www.drugs.com/pregnancy/sodium-nitrite-sodium-thiosulfate.html

http://www.environmentalhealthnews.org/ehs/newscience/2013/06/nitrate-in-moms-drinking-water/

http://www.sixwise.com/newsletters/07/08/22/the-dangers-of-nitrites-the-foods-they-are-found-in-and-why-you-want-to-avoid-them.htm

http://www.sixwise.com/newsletters/06/04/05/12_dangerous_food_additives_the_dirty_dozen_food_additives_you_really_need_to_be_aware_of.htm

http://saveourbones.com/osteoporosis-milk-myth/

http://www.pcrm.org/health/diets/vegdiets/health-concerns-about-dairy-products

http://www.healthguidance.org/entry/9973/1/Negative-Effects-of-Dairy-Products.html

https://webndbitesoflife.wordpress.com/tag/dairy-and-its-effects-on-health/

http://www.wisegeek.com/what-is-processed-cheese.htm

http://www.mirror.co.uk/news/weird-news/whats-processed-cheese-slices-shock-5022840

https://birthdefects.org/aspartame-2/

http://www.huffingtonpost.ca/2013/04/17/worst-toxic-food-ingredients_n_3101043.html

http://www.digitaljournal.com/life/health/chemicals-used-in-packaging-processed-foods-may-be-harmful/article/372101

http://www.naturalnews.com/027969_processed_foods_chemicals.html#

http://www.eatingwell.com/food_news_origins/food_news/the_hidden_health_risks_of_food_dyes

http://www.foodsafetynews.com/2010/07/popular-food-dyes-linked-to-cancer-adhd-and-allergies/#.VkESLDZdFPY

http://ncsoy.org/media-resources/history-of-soybeans/

http://www.soyfoods.org/press-releases/soyfoods-are-part-of-americas-history

http://healthyeating.sfgate.com/eating-soy-increase-estrogen-production-2870.html

http://www.ncbi.nlm.nih.gov/pubmed/23752918

http://www.second-opinions.co.uk/soy-online-service/04birthdefects.htm#.VkEmcjZdFPY

http://articles.mercola.com/sites/articles/archive/2000/02/06/vegetarian-pregnancy.aspx

http://www.westonaprice.org/health-topics/effects-of-antenatal-exposure-to-phytoestrogens-on-human-male-reproductive-and-urogenital-development/

http://naturalsociety.com/genetically-modified-foods/

http://www.webmd.com/food-recipes/truth-about-gmos

http://www.disabled-world.com/fitness/gm-foods.php

http://www.alternet.org/personal-health/genetically-engineered-soybeans-give-altered-milk-and-stunted-offspring-researchers

http://www.naturalnews.com/051854_genetically_modified_soybeans_stunted_growth_breast_milk_deficiency.html

http://articles.mercola.com/sites/articles/archive/2012/05/13/ge-food-cause-birth-defects.aspx#!

http://www.webmd.com/diet/guide/understanding-trans-fats

http://www.mayoclinic.org/diseases-conditions/high-blood-cholesterol/in-depth/trans-fat/ART-20046114?pg=1

http://www.heart.org/HEARTORG/GettingHealthy/NutritionCenter/HealthyEating/Trans-Fats_UCM_301120_Article.jsp#.VkJJbTZdFPY

http://www.fda.gov/Food/PopularTopics/ucm292278.htm

http://www.cnn.com/2015/06/16/health/fda-trans-fat/index.html

http://www.hsph.harvard.edu/nutritionsource/transfats/

http://www.empr.com/news/eating-more-trans-fats-bad-for-memory/article/421044/

http://www.ncbi.nlm.nih.gov/pmc/articles/PMC3192475/

http://www.medscape.com/medline/abstract/20650350

http://www.foodnavigator-usa.com/R-D/Trans-fat-consumption-during-pregnancy-linked-to-higher-birth-weights

http://www.webmd.com/men/features/exercise-benefits

http://www.cdc.gov/physicalactivity/basics/pa-health/index.htm

http://health.usnews.com/health-news/diet-fitness/slideshows/7-mind-blowing-benefits-of-exercise

http://www.mayoclinic.org/healthy-lifestyle/fitness/in-depth/exercise/art-20048389

http://www.cdc.gov/physicalactivity/basics/adults/index.htm

http://www.heart.org/HEARTORG/GettingHealthy/PhysicalActivity/StartWalking/American-Heart-Association-Guidelines_UCM_307976_Article.jsp#.VkKQxTZdFPY

http://www.who.int/dietphysicalactivity/factsheet_adults/en/

http://www.fitnessmagazine.com/health/pregnancy/how-exercise-affects-fertility/

http://www.webmd.com/baby/news/20120315/trying-to-get-pregnant-moderate-exercise-may-help

http://www.carolinaconceptions.com/fertility101/exercise-and-fertility/

http://americanpregnancy.org/pregnancy-health/exercise-during-pregnancy/

http://www.webmd.com/baby/guide/exercise-during-pregnancy

http://www.whattoexpect.com/pregnancy/exercise-benefits

http://www.fitpregnancy.com/exercise/prenatal-workouts/33-reasons-exercise-now

http://www.prevention.com/health/healthy-living/benefits-exercise-during-pregnancy-baby

http://www.pregnancyexercise.co.nz/exercising-during-pregnancy-benefits-for-your-baby/

http://www.webmd.com/baby/exercise-during-pregnancy

http://www.webmd.com/infertility-and-reproduction/news/20071211/obesity-linked-to-infertility-in-women

http://www.calculator.net/bmi-calculator.html

http://www.news-medical.net/health/Obesity-and-Infertility.aspx

http://www.webmd.com/infertility-and-reproduction/news/20041022/obesity-takes-toll-on-sperm-fertility

http://attainfertility.com/article/sleep-infertility-link

http://www.huffingtonpost.com/2013/10/18/sleep-fertility_n_4122829.html

http://www.fertility-health.com/effects-of-sleep-deprivation.html

http://www.webmd.com/baby/features/drinking-alcohol-during-pregnancy

http://www.cdc.gov/ncbddd/fasd/alcohol-use.html

http://www.marchofdimes.org/pregnancy/alcohol-during-pregnancy.aspx

http://americanpregnancy.org/pregnancy-health/pregnancy-and-alcohol/

http://www.euro.who.int/en/data-and-evidence/evidence-informed-policy-making/publications/hen-summaries-of-network-members-reports/is-low-dose-alcohol-exposure-during-pregnancy-harmful

http://blog.sfgate.com/sfmoms/2009/04/01/pregnant-european-women-drink-right/

http://newsfeed.time.com/2013/04/18/light-drinking-during-pregnancy-is-not-harmful-for-baby-study-says/

http://www.fertility-health.com/infertility-and-alcohol.html

https://www.fertilityauthority.com/articles/alcohol-and-fertility

http://www.cdc.gov/reproductivehealth/MaternalInfantHealth/TobaccoUsePregnancy/index.htm

http://attainfertility.com/article/smoking-infertility

http://www.ncbi.nlm.nih.gov/pmc/articles/PMC2040350/

http://www.livestrong.com/article/172303-long-term-effects-of-tobacco-on-a-fetus/

http://americanpregnancy.org/pregnancy-health/smoking-during-pregnancy/

http://www.babycenter.com/0_how-smoking-during-pregnancy-affects-you-and-your-baby_1405720.bc?page=1

http://www.mayoclinic.org/healthy-lifestyle/adult-health/in-depth/secondhand-smoke/art-20043914?pg=2

http://www.nbcnews.com/id/35318118/ns/health-addictions/t/third-hand-smoke-danger-babies-toddlers/#.Vku5yTZdFPY

http://blogs.babycenter.com/mom_stories/third-hand-smoke-is-a-hazard-to-babys-health/

http://www.scientificamerican.com/article/what-is-third-hand-smoke/

http://www.marchofdimes.org/pregnancy/smoking-during-pregnancy.aspx

http://www.babycentre.co.uk/a541318/illegal-drugs-in-pregnancy

http://www.conceiveeasy.com/get-pregnant/illegal-drugs-and-their-affect-on-your-fertility/

http://www.vice.com/read/we-asked-three-doctors-how-illegal-drugs-affect-your-pregnancy-101

http://www.thegooddrugsguide.com/getreal/drug-babies-and-the-effects-of-drug-abuse-during-pregnancy.htm

http://fetal-exposure.org/the-effects-of-hallucinogen-use-during-pregnancy

https://www.fertilityauthority.com/articles/effects-caffeine-fertility

http://www.resolve.org/about-infertility/optimizing-fertility/caffeine-does-it-affect-your-fertility-and-pregnancy.html

http://www.mayoclinic.org/healthy-lifestyle/nutrition-and-healthy-eating/in-depth/caffeine/art-20049372?pg=1

http://www.starbucks.com/search?keywords=caffeine+content

http://www.livestrong.com/article/1002655-prenatal-development-caffeine/

http://americanpregnancy.org/pregnancy-health/caffeine-during-pregnancy/

http://www.psychiatry.emory.edu/PROGRAMS/GADrug/caffeine.htm

http://www.ncbi.nlm.nih.gov/pubmed/20427730

http://www.ncbi.nlm.nih.gov/pmc/articles/PMC2753720/

http://pediatrics.aappublications.org/content/130/2/e305.long

http://www.tandfonline.com/doi/abs/10.3109/00207458808985738

http://www.cabdirect.org/abstracts/19911434740.html;jsessionid=A3B375DC1A1BA19F1A40B2C73A4F16FF

http://tipsdiscover.com/health/neurodevelopmental-consequences-coffeecaffeine-exposure/

http://www.cdc.gov/ncbddd/adhd/data.html

http://www.webmd.com/diet/what-to-know-about-omega-3s-and-fish?page=4

http://www.webmd.com/healthy-aging/omega-3-fatty-acids-fact-sheet

http://www.sciencedaily.com/releases/2008/04/080409110029.htm

http://www.mayoclinic.org/drugs-supplements/vitamin-c/background/HRB-20060322

http://www.naturalmedicines.therapeuticresearch.com

http://www.babycenter.com/0_folic-acid-why-you-need-it-before-and-during-pregnancy_476.bc

http://www.healthline.com/health-slideshow/surprising-benefits-probiotics

http://www.foodmatters.tv/articles-1/6-healing-benefits-of-probiotics

http://fertilitynj.com/infertility/female-infertility/genetic-causes/

http://ghr.nlm.nih.gov/gene/MTHFR

http://mthfr.net/

https://madeinamericathebook.wordpress.com/2011/09/21/breastfeeding-history/

http://www.huffingtonpost.com/2013/02/07/breastfeeding-rate-has-in_n_2639043.html

http://www.ncbi.nlm.nih.gov/pmc/articles/PMC2684040/

http://www.surgeongeneral.gov/library/calls/breastfeeding/factsheet.html

http://www.womenshealth.gov/breastfeeding/breastfeeding-benefits.html

http://www.who.int/features/factfiles/breastfeeding/en/

http://www.cwsglobal.org/blog/benefits-of-breastfeeding.html

http://www.medicaldaily.com/9-toxic-chemicals-found-furniture-your-home-hazard-zone-256572

http://blackdoctor.org/14220/toxic-chemicals-in-furniture/

http://www.sfgate.com/health/article/Warning-on-chemicals-in-children-s-furniture-4994841.php

http://www.oprah.com/health/Are-Toxins-in-Your-Furniture-Making-You-Sick

http://www.green-talk.com/are-toxic-chemicals-lurking-in-your-furniture-and-building-products/

http://www.ehow.com/list_5818265_list-mattress-chemicals.html

http://web.archive.org/web/20001026033455/http://www.sids.org.uk/fsid/limerick.htm

http://www.dispatch.com/content/stories/national_world/2012/12/29/baby-mattresses-found-to-be-toxic.html

http://www.foxnews.com/health/2014/04/02/crib-mattresses-release-potentially-harmful-chemicals-study-finds.html

http://www.naturalnews.com/001061.html

http://articles.mercola.com/sites/articles/archive/2011/12/21/are-you-slowly-killing-your-family-with-hidden-dioxane-in-your-laundry-detergent.aspx

http://www.huffingtonpost.com/2012/04/26/tide-detergent-1-4-dioxane_n_1455575.html

http://www.abc.net.au/news/2014-05-08/cancer-jean-risk/5438614

http://www.recallowl.com/recalls/toxic

http://www.king5.com/story/tech/science/aerospace/2014/08/04/13282784/

http://awesomebeginnings4children.com/the-harmful-chemicals-in-disposable-diapers/

http://www.livestrong.com/article/111348-chemicals-disposable-diapers/

http://www.cbc.ca/news/technology/disposable-diapers-are-they-dangerous-1.888074

http://www.nrdc.org/living/healthreports/hidden-hazards-air-fresheners.asp

http://www.scientificamerican.com/article/nontoxic-air-fresheners/

http://www.care2.com/greenliving/exposed-cancer-causing-toxins-found-in-air-fresheners.html

http://www.keeperofthehome.org/2012/04/toxins-in-candles-sad-but-true.html

http://www.greenamerica.org/livinggreen/candles.cfm

http://wellnessmama.com/22656/dont-use-scented-candles/

http://healthland.time.com/2009/08/19/chemicals_in_candles/

http://www.abc15.com/news/national/can-burning-candles-make-you-sick-university-studies-scrutinize-possible-release-of-toxic-fumes

http://www.pesticideinfo.org/Detail_Chemical.jsp?Rec_Id=PC34054

http://brooklynherborium.com/2013/03/19/whats-wrong-with-vaseline/

http://health-report.co.uk/petroleum_petrolatum_health_concerns.htm

http://health-report.co.uk/harmful_toxic_toiletries_chemicals_cancer_causing.html

http://www.cancer.org/cancer/cancercauses/othercarcinogens/athome/talcum-powder-and-cancer

http://www.webmd.com/ovarian-cancer/news/20000411/talc-powder-ovarian-cancer-link

http://articles.mercola.com/sites/articles/archive/2008/10/14/talcum-powder-linked-to-ovarian-cancer.aspx#!

http://www.cbsnews.com/news/baby-wipe-chemical-tied-to-allergic-reactions-in-some-kids/

http://www.dailymail.co.uk/health/article-2538668/The-horrific-damage-BABY-WIPES-childrens-skin-Chemical-wipes-cause-itchy-red-rash.html

http://www.ecolife.com/parenting/organic-baby-body/baby-care-product-chemicals.html

http://www.naturalnews.com/001586.html

http://www2.epa.gov/insect-repellents/deet

http://www.popsci.com/article/science/deet-safe-use

http://healthresearchfunding.org/dangers-deet/

http://www.scientificamerican.com/article/is-it-true-that-the-deet/

http://nj.gov/health/eoh/rtkweb/documents/fs/0765.pdf

http://www.thedermreview.com/octinoxate/

http://www.womenshealthmag.com/beauty/6-scary-sunscreen-ingredients-and-6-safe-spf-products

http://www.ecomall.com/greenshopping/cosmetic.htm

http://enhs.umn.edu/current/5103/phth/harmful.html

http://grinningplanet.com/2005/10-04/triclosan-article.htm

http://www.fda.gov/ForConsumers/ConsumerUpdates/ucm205999.htm

http://www.mayoclinic.org/healthy-lifestyle/adult-health/expert-answers/triclosan/faq-20057861

http://www.thedermreview.com/triethanolamine/

http://www.ewg.org/skindeep/ingredient/706639/TRIETHANOLAMINE/

http://www.top10homeremedies.com/kitchen-ingredients/10-health-benefits-of-drinking-water.html

http://www.fitday.com/fitness-articles/nutrition/healthy-eating/5-little-known-benefits-of-drinking-water.html

http://www.webmd.com/diet/6-reasons-to-drink-water

https://www.organicfacts.net/health-benefits/other/health-benefits-of-drinking-water.html

http://womeninbalance.org/2012/10/26/xenoestrogens-what-are-they-how-to-avoid-them/

https://endojourney.wordpress.com/2009/07/31/a-list-of-xenoestrogens/

http://www.womenlivingnaturally.com/articlepage.php?id=73

http://www.healthguidance.org/entry/14913/1/What-Chemicals-Are-in-Tap-Water.html

http://www2.epa.gov/dwstandardsregulations

http://ezinearticles.com/?The-Five-Most-Harmful-Chemicals-Found-in-Tap-Water&id=2027700

http://articles.mercola.com/sites/articles/archive/2013/12/28/fluoride-drinking-water.aspx

Made in the USA
San Bernardino, CA
03 December 2017